THE EASY AIP DIET COOKBOOK

TABLE OF CONTENTS

INTRODUCTION

Thank you for the purchase of *The Easy AIP Diet Cookbook: Delicious Autoimmune Paleo Recipes for Healing, Includes a 30-Day Meal Plan with Nourishing Allergen-Free Meals*. This book contains detailed information about the autoimmune protocol as well as easy and nourishing recipes you can easily make in your own kitchen.

Autoimmune Protocol is a holistic approach that comprises a diet-based system and a healthy lifestyle approach to correct autoimmune diseases. AIP focuses on supplementing the body with a nutrient-rich diet and embracing a healthy lifestyle to help the body in chronic disease management. Subscribing to the autoimmune protocol helps to address gut health issues, inflammation, hormone regulation, and generally improve the immune system. There are three stages in the Autoimmune protocol diet-approach. These include the elimination stage, the reintroduction stage, and the maintenance stage.

Elimination Stage: This is the first stage in the healing process where foods that cause gut irritation and aid imbalances in the immune system are eliminated. The foods that are eliminated are replaced with nutrient-rich foods that help in the healing process. The AIP diet modification is a strict approach meant to be followed for a certain period of time (about 30 – 60 days) until there is a reduction in the symptoms, and the body's health is restored. Foods such as eggs, nightshade vegetables, alcohol, processed foods, etc. are eliminated while foods such as fermented vegetables, coconut oil, avocado oil, leafy greens, glycine-rich foods, etc. are introduced into the daily diet. It is essential to complement the introduction of nutrient-dense foods with a healthy lifestyle practice to get the best out of the autoimmune protocol.

Reintroduction Stage: This is the next stage after completing the first stage for the recommended period of time. It is also crucial at this stage to be strategic and careful when reintroducing foods back into the daily diet. It is advisable to introduce one food per time and give time to study how the body reacts to the food before adding another food.

Maintenance Stage: This is the last stage of the diet approach, which involves maintenance through healthy eating and living. It is at this stage each person gets to design and develop a personal roadmap towards better health.

The Easy AIP Diet Cookbook provides you with simple, nutritious and tasty recipes that will help speed up the healing of your autoimmune condition. The AIP recipes provided in this cookbook combine easy-to-find ingredients with quick prep and cook times to enable spend less time in the kitchen. All the recipes provided do not include any grains, egg, nightshades, nuts, seeds, soy, beans etc.

With loads of wholesome recipes, you'll find lots of choices for any meal of the day in this cookbook. The *Easy AIP Diet Cookbook* is packed with healing, restorative recipes to repair your gut and restore proper immune function.

CHAPTER 1: ABOUT AIP

The Autoimmune Protocol (AIP), also known as the paleo autoimmune protocol, is a form of elimination diet used in chronic disease management, which involves providing the body with nutritional supplements designed to regulate the hormones, heal leaky gut and reduce inflammation. The autoimmune protocol helps to avoid processed food with inflammatory compounds and also goes beyond the dietary framework to encourage living a healthy lifestyle. There are usually three lifestyle factors considered as healthy living; these include: getting sufficient sleep, stress management, and staying active. They are crucial for gut health and are also modulators of hormones and immune functions.

The Autoimmune Protocol is aimed at eliminating symptoms created by autoimmune diseases or disorders. An autoimmune disorder is a situation where one's immune system wrongly attacks healthy cells in one's body. While the immune system is known to protect the body against attacks; in the case of autoimmune disorders, the immune

11

system finds it difficult to identify between one's body cells and foreign invaders. As a result, it wrongly takes part of the body as foreign invaders and sends autoantibodies to attack the cells. Examples of autoimmune disorders include type 1 diabetes - which affects the pancreas, thyroiditis - which attacks the thyroid gland, etc. Some other autoimmune diseases do not affect only one part of the body but affect multiple organs and sometimes even the entire body; an example is the systemic lupus erythematosus, which affects the whole body. Researchers are yet to find what exactly causes autoimmune disorders, and it is probably the reason there is yet to be a known medical curative treatment for them; however, studies revolve around diet, infections, genetics, etc. AIP, therefore, focuses on eliminating food contents that aid autoimmune disorders and are considered detrimental to health as the case may be.

It is worthy of note that sometimes, the food contents eliminated are not exactly harmful in themselves, but as long as the contents are not in alignment with the goal of AIP, they are considered detrimental. The main goal of AIP is to supply nutrients to the body and, at the same time, ensure that no food or food content is interfering with the healing process. The dietary supplement alone is not enough to reverse the symptoms caused by autoimmune diseases; this is why AIP promotes the dietary supplements together with the healthy lifestyle practice. When there is enough sleep, activeness, and the stress level is well monitored, it aids a healthy gut microbial environment. However, in the quest to be active, it is essential to avoid overtraining as this may increase the permeability of the intestine.

Pros and Cons of Autoimmune Protocol

The disadvantages associated with the AIP diet include: how it interferes with the day to day activities, having to learn how to cook since the rest of the family will be eating something different, and also how some of the meals are expensive to prepare and requires a lot of organization.

While those may be con reasons against autoimmune protocol, the sacrifice is usually well worth it. As a result, most people (especially those with autoimmune conditions) find that the benefits of AIP indeed outweigh the required sacrifice. There is always no price too high to pay for perfect health.

The pros and benefits of following the AIP diet include but not limited to: how the diet helps to reduce inflammation and reverse the symptoms of autoimmune disorders, how the diet helps the body to operate at its best, and how it also helps to address the gut dysfunction situation.

Following the strict diet may be overwhelming at first, but one soon finds that the benefits truly outweigh the burdens of its restrictions. It is crucial for a person with autoimmune disease to be completely committed to the diet if the symptoms are going to be reversed.

CHAPTER 2: THE BASICS OF AIP

The basics of the Autoimmune Protocol borders around a diet-based approach to eliminate inflammation caused by autoimmune diseases. Ultimately, it is essential to strictly follow the AIP eating plan for a few weeks before reintroducing foods outside of the AIP diet. The autoimmune protocol diet goal is to remove foods that could trigger inflammation or affect the gut and replace those foods with nutrient-dense food that aids and promotes health. By following the restrictive diet and using it as medicine addresses the underlying hormonal imbalances by reducing inflammation and healing the damaged gut barrier, causing the immune system to respond. Understanding the concept of gut dysfunction is fundamental to understanding why the Autoimmune Protocol works in stimulating the immune system. Gut dysfunction or leaky gut is simply the breakdown of the intestinal lining, creating small holes in the intestines. Foods are released through these small holes to the rest of the body, and hence, it triggers the immune system to respond. The signs of leaky guts include digestive issues, hormonal imbalances, food allergies, autoimmune conditions, etc. AIP diets work impressively to correct these conditions, but as stated earlier, it is essential to follow the strict eating plan for several weeks.

What to avoid and what to eat on the AIP diet

In order to stay on track and prevent interference with the healing process, it's crucial to know the foods to avoid and the foods that can be eaten on the AIP diet.

Grains: You should avoid all forms of grains – rice, millet, oats, wheat, etc.

Vegetables: You should also avoid nightshades vegetables – tomatoes, eggplant, onion, white potatoes, goji berries, and peppery spices. You are free to eat every other vegetable – cabbage, cauliflower, cucumber, asparagus, sweet potatoes, leafy greens, etc.

Meats: Factory-farmed meats and farm-raised seafood are not permitted on the AIP diet, but it is okay to eat beef, chicken, bison, turkey, wild-caught fish, etc.

Legumes: You should avoid Peanuts, soy, and all kinds of beans except for snap peas and string beans. You may eat haricot vert, snap peas, string beans, etc.

Eggs: Avoid all kinds of eggs with no exception.

Fruits: You may eat all kinds of fruits. The diet encourages the daily intake of fruits but should be kept to a minimum (about one to two pieces per day) to stabilize blood sugar level and avoid irritating the gut.

Dairy: Coconut milk without additives is permitted. But cheese, yogurt, ice cream should be avoided.

Nuts and Seeds: You should stay away from nuts and seeds – almonds, chia seeds, cashews, cacao, etc. You can have teas that are not seed-based such as green tea and black tea.

Fats: You should avoid butter, ghee, canola oil, margarine, and other seed oils in your diet. Only eat olive oil, avocado oil, fat, avocado etc.

Sugar: You should stay away from sugars. Small portions of honey or maple syrup are permitted.

Fermented foods: Fermented soy products should be avoided. Kombucha, kimchi, etc. are permitted.

Nonsteroidal Anti-inflammatory Drugs (NSAIDs): All NSAIDs – Ibuprofen, ketorolac, etc. are not permitted on the AIP diet.

Food Additives: You should avoid all forms of food additives – guar gum, nitrates, aspartame, benzoic acid, etc.

Alcohol: All kinds of alcohol should be avoided – beer, extracts, liquor, etc.

Staying away from these foods may be overwhelming for starters, but remembering the purpose of staying away is a great motivation to abide and follow the strict eating plan for the set time. Although, how long you choose to stay on the AIP diet is completely up to you, it's recommended to follow the diet-based approach for a minimum of 30 – 60 days. Many other people choose to stay on the diet until they see positive changes in their autoimmune conditions.

Basically, the AIP diet helps to remove all toxins and gut irritants, and then replace them with food contents that aid healing of the leaky gut. With rich supplements embedded in the diet, it repairs damaged organs and restores digestive enzymes, healthy bacteria (probiotics), hydrochloric acid, and soluble fiber back into the body system. The AIP diet is not a lifetime treatment for autoimmune disorders; however, after following the strict eating plan for the recommended weeks, it's expected that you start reintroducing foods outside of the AIP diet into your eating plan. It is important to do so one at a time. For instance, you may first introduce grains like oats back into your eating plan but wait for about 72 hours to see how your body reacts to the food. Other things to pay attention to when reintroducing foods outside on the AIP diet include; digestion, bloating, cognitive function, mood, etc. You can then make decisions based on your level of progress. AIP diet is a very strict diet-approach, but it works impressively, and the benefits outweigh the sacrifice involved.

CHAPTER 3: AUTOIMMUNE DIET FOOD LIST

FOODS ALLOWED ON THE AUTOIMMUNE PROTOCOL DIET

Fruits

Fruits are rich in fiber, and most of them contain antioxidants that help to shield body cells from damage. However, fruits should not be over-consumed and about two servings a day is recommended;

Citrus

Cherry

Berries

Watermelon

Pomegranate

Pear

Peach

Melons

Mango

Pineapple

Plum

Persimmon

Banana

Avocado

Apricot

Apple

Kiwi

Grape

Fig

Date

Coconut

Vegetables

Vegetables are loaded with fiber and phytonutrients that enable the human body to thrive! About nine servings of vegetables a day are recommended;

Cauliflower

Carrots

Cabbage

Bok Choy

Spinach

Avocado

Asparagus

Arugula

Parsnip

Onion

Kale

Jicama

Fennel

Cucumber

Chard

Brussels

Mushroom

Sweet potato

Squash

Lettuce

Leek

Broccoli

Beets

Artichoke

Proteins

Animal protein that is of high-quality animal protein gives healthy fats, minerals, and adequate energy. The AIP diet endorses animal protein as a healthful food. Therefore, high-quality options such as wild-caught, pasture-raised, and grass-fed are to be consumed when possible;

Fish

Duck

Chicken

Venison

Turkey

Shellfish

Lamb

Bison

Beef

Bone broth & organ meats

Herbs

Herbs contain fiber and phytonutrients that are great for our bodies. Below is a list of herbs and spices that are autoimmune-friendly;

Turmeric

Thyme

Sage

Cinnamon

Cilantro

Chives

Bay leaf

Basil

Saffron

Rosemary

Peppermint

Parsley

Mint

Garlic

Ginger

Dill

Fats

Healthy fats are great for the body as they help to control the inflammation process in the body. They are the carriers of nutrients, and they help us to stay satisfied. Healthy fats are incredibly essential to be included in every meal to aid the healing process of the body and to keep you full;

Palm oil

Avocado oil

Olive oil

Coconut oil

Chicken fat

Beef tallow

Pantry Staples

Honey

Dried fruit

Coconut sugar

Tigernut flour

Tapioca starch

Arrowroot starch

Coconut flour

Cassava flour

Carob powder

FOODS NOT ALLOWED ON THE AUTOIMMUNE PROTOCOL DIET

All Eggs

One of the most common allergens are eggs, and they easily irritate the gut. The whites are more irritating than the yolks, so most individuals are able to reintroduce egg yolks effortlessly than whole eggs.

Grains and Gluten

Autoimmune patients also suffer from a leaky gut. Grains and gluten can cause leaky gut (or intestinal permeability), and it is vital to avoid them to enable quick healing of the body;

Buckwheat

Wheat

Sorghum

Rice

Quinoa

Oat

Millet

Corn

Bulger

Rye

Barley

Amaranth

Legumes

Legumes such as beans can be harmful to the lining of the gut and should be avoided to promote healing;

Soybeans

Peanuts

Lima beans

Lentils

Kidney beans

Fava beans

Chickpeas

Black beans

Seed and Berry Spices

Seed spices can be inflammatory to the lining of the gut. So, avoid them for quick healing;

Poppy Seeds

Black Pepper

Nutmeg

Mustard

Fennel seed

Cumin

Celery seed

Caraway

Anise

Allspice

Seeds and Nuts

Seeds and nuts can cause inflammation in the gut lining.

Cashew

Canola

Walnut

Pine nuts

Pecan

Hemp

Hazelnut

Sunflower

Sesame

Safflower

Chia

Brazil nut

Almond

Pumpkin

Pistachio

Flax

Cocoa

Coffee

<u>Dairy</u>

Dairy can trigger inflammation and allergies. They can also harm the gut lining; so, they should be avoided while on this diet. However, high-quality dairy can be taken moderately for after healing;

Yogurt

Milk

Ghee

Cream

Cheese

Butter

Nightshades

The nightshades are the kinds of vegetables that can stimulate inflammation, particularly in individuals with joint issues;

All red spices

All peppers (bell pepper, spicy pepper, etc.)

Tomatillo

Tomato

Potato

Eggplant

Ground cherries

Goji Berries

<u>Sugar and Additives</u>

Sugars and other additives such as food dyes and gums do not aid healing. However, natural sweeteners like coconut sugar, maple syrup, and honey can be used moderately.

<u>Alcohol</u>

Alcohol does not stimulate healing. But you can take them moderately after healing has taken place.

CHAPTER 4: 30-DAY AUTOIMMUNE DIET MEAL PLAN

This 30-day meal plan will help get you started on the Autoimmune diet. The recipes for each meal can be found in this book.

Day 1

Breakfast: Brussels Sprout Coleslaw

Lunch: Coconut Turmeric Balls

Dinner: Barbeque Buns

Day 2

Breakfast: Ramen Noodle Soup

Lunch: Sweet Potato Skins (Stuffed)

Dinner: Green Salad with Italian Dressing

Day 3

Breakfast: Carrot Banana Bread N'Oatmeal

Lunch: Chicken Tenders

Dinner: Roasted Vegetable with Dressing

Day 4

Breakfast: Pumpkin Pancakes

Lunch: Lime Cilantro Cauliflower

Dinner: Lemon Tuna Salad

Day 5

Breakfast: AIP-Friendly Granola

Lunch: Steak Salad with Tarragon Dressing

Dinner: Notato Salad with dressing

Day 6

Breakfast: Avocado Chicken Salad

Lunch: Lemon Tuna Salad

Dinner: Meatballs with Nomato Sauce

Day 7

Breakfast: Avocado Kale Salad with Strawberry

Lunch: Melon Salad

Dinner: Slow-cooked Duck Breast

Day 8

Breakfast: Zucchini Noodle

Lunch: Baby Artichokes

Dinner: Sashimi Salad

Day 9

Breakfast: Warm Porridge with Lemon

Lunch: Roasted Leek Greens

Dinner: Seaweed Salad

Day 10

Breakfast: Chicken and Tarragon Sausage

Lunch: Mushroom Turnip Greens with Almonds

Dinner: Rosemary and Pears Roasted Chicken

Day 11

Breakfast: Avocado Fries

Lunch: Carrot Cilantro Mash

Dinner: Elk Meatloaf with Apple & Sage

Day 12

Breakfast: Garlic Kale Chips

Lunch: Balsamic-Sauced Chicken Livers with Grapes

Dinner: Smoked Salmon Ceviche

Day 13

Breakfast: Vegetable Scramble

Lunch: Dairy-free Alfredo Chicken

Dinner: Barbeque Buns

Day 14

Breakfast: Shrimp Fried Cauliflower Rice

Lunch: Oyster Sauerkraut Soup

Dinner: Green Salad with Italian Dressing

Day 15

Breakfast: Ambrosia Salad

Lunch: Shrimp Fried Cauliflower Rice

Dinner: Roasted Vegetable with Dressing

Day 16

Breakfast: Waffles with Pumpkin Spice

Lunch: Coconut Shrimp and Grits

Dinner: Lemon Tuna Salad

Day 17

Breakfast: Coconut Cassava Pancakes

Lunch: Salmon Nori Wrap

Dinner: Notato Salad with dressing

Day 18

Breakfast: Ramen Noodle Soup

Lunch: Nomato-sauced Shrimp

Dinner: Meatballs with Nomato Sauce

Day 19

Breakfast: Carrot Banana Bread N'Oatmeal

Lunch: Chocolate-like Cookies

Dinner: Slow-cooked Duck Breast

Day 20

Breakfast: Pumpkin Pancakes

Lunch: Waffles with Pumpkin Spice

Dinner: Sashimi Salad

Day 21

Breakfast: AIP-Friendly Granola

Lunch: Coconut Turmeric Balls

Dinner: Smoked Salmon Ceviche

Day 22

Breakfast: Avocado Chicken Salad

Lunch: Sweet Potato Skins (Stuffed)

Dinner: AIP-Friendly Ceviche

Day 23

Breakfast: Brussels Sprout Coleslaw

Lunch: Chicken Tenders

Dinner: Oyster Sauerkraut Soup

Day 24

Breakfast: Avocado Kale Salad with Strawberry

Lunch: Lime Cilantro Cauliflower

Dinner: Dairy-free Alfredo Chicken

Day 25

Breakfast: Zucchini Noodle

Lunch: Steak Salad with Tarragon Dressing

Dinner: Rosemary and Pears Roasted Chicken

Day 26

Breakfast: Warm Porridge with Lemon

Lunch: Lemon Tuna Salad

Dinner: Carbonara Spaghetti Squash

Day 27

Breakfast: Chicken and Tarragon Sausage

Lunch: Roasted Leek Greens

Dinner: Shallots Lamb Roast with Golden Beets

Day 28

Breakfast: Garlic Kale Chips

Lunch: Carrot Cilantro Mash

Dinner: Balsamic-Sauced Chicken Livers with Grapes

Day 29

Breakfast: Shrimp Fried Cauliflower Rice

Lunch: Nomato-sauced Shrimp

Dinner: Melon Salad

Day 30

Breakfast: Waffles with Pumpkin Spice

Lunch: Coconut Shrimp Lime

Dinner: Steak Salad with Tarragon Dressing

CHAPTER 5: BREAKFAST RECIPES

With all the restrictions on the Autoimmune Protocol diet, breakfast may start to seem like the hardest meal to prepare, but it is not as it looks if you are adventurous. Here are a few breakfast recipes you can make quickly and enjoy.

RAMEN NOODLE SOUP

Yield: 4 serves

Cook Time: 15 minutes

Ingredients

- 5 oz. of smoked turkey bacon
- 3 carrots
- 1 teaspoon of mild unflavored coconut oil
- 3 chicken breasts

- 15 mushrooms (chestnut-brown)
- ½ teaspoon of ground ginger
- 3 cups of chicken broth
- 2 large Zucchini
- Sea salt (about a pinch)
- Spinach (2 handfuls)
- Cilantro
- 3 onions (green)

Instructions

- Cut the chicken into thin slices. Prepare the mushrooms, cleanse thoroughly and slice. Also, peel the carrots and slice.
- Prepare a large saucepan and apply heat (averagely) to it.
- Add coconut oil and the turkey bacon, and allow it to cook gently until it sizzles and appears to turn golden.
- Then, add the sliced mushrooms and carrots to the saucepan with ground ginger and stir well. Then, stir in the chicken slices.
- Add the chicken broth and a pinch of salt. Stir the mix and allow it to simmer for about 5 minutes. In the meantime, prepare your zucchini into noodles.

- When the chicken is cooked, add the zucchini noodles and 2 handfuls of spinach to the saucepan and stir together.
- Allow cooking for about 2 – 3 minutes. Then, slice the green onions to the mix and stir together.
- While the recipe is ready to be served, wash the cilantro and cut into smaller bunches.
- Divide the recipe between four serving bowls, pour the extra broth over the contents of each bowl and top with cilantro.

Nutrition Facts: Calories – 448, Protein – 44.6g, Total Fat – 21.3g, Saturated Fat – 8.6g, Cholesterol – 93mg, Total Sugars – 10.3g, Dietary Fiber – 5.5g, Total Carbohydrate – 20.9g, Iron – 5mg, Potassium – 1337mg, Calcium – 85mg, Vitamin D – 243mcg.

CARROT BANANA BREAD N'OATMEAL

Cook Time: 1 hour 10 minutes

Yield: 7 Serves

Ingredients

- 2 (10 oz.) bags of shredded carrots
- 13½ oz. can of coconut milk, full fat
- ½ tsp of baking soda
- 2 tsp of ground cinnamon
- 1 tsp of fine sea salt
- 1 cup of mashed yellow banana
- ¾ cup of shredded coconut (unsweetened)
- ¼ cup of coconut flour
- ½ cup of raisins

Instructions

- Heat the oven to a temperature of about 350 ºF.
- Prepare a large mixing bowl and mix all the ingredients in it until they are evenly mixed.
- Transfer the mix into a 9 by 13 inches glass casserole dish and use a spatula to hold down firmly.

- Cover securely and bake for 55 minutes. Allow cooling for 5 minutes before serving.

- Top with more raisins or coconut, if preferred.

Nutrition Facts: Calories – 286, Protein – 3.9g, Total Fat – 16.4g, Saturated fat – 14.4g, Total Carbohydrates – 37.4g, Dietary Fiber – 8.6g, Total Sugars – 22.4g, Iron – 3mg, Potassium – 371mg, Calcium – 40mg, Cholesterol – 0mg, Sodium – 463mg.

PUMPKIN PANCAKES

Cook Time: 30 minutes

Yield: 8 serves

Ingredients

- 3/4 cup of canned pumpkin puree
- $1^1/_3$ cups of cassava flour
- 1½ teaspoons of pumpkin pie spice
- 1/2 teaspoon of baking soda
- ½ cup of coconut sugar
- 1 tablespoon gelatin
- 3 tablespoons of hot water
- ¾ cup of coconut or tiger-nut milk
- ¼ cup of coconut oil (melted)
- ¼ cup of maple syrup
- 2 teaspoons of vanilla

Instructions

- Prepare a large mixing bowl and add cassava flour, baking soda, pumpkin spice, coconut sugar to it. Whisk together.

- In another mixing bowl, add pumpkin puree, coconut oil, vanilla, maple syrup, coconut, or tiger-nut milk and mix to combine.

- Combine gelatin with one tablespoon of cold water in a small bowl and continuously stir until uniform. Add two tablespoons of hot water and stir until the gelatin is dissolved. Stir into the mixing bowl that contains the wet ingredients.

- Carefully add the wet ingredients to the dry and stir gently.

- Place a large saucepan over medium heat and spray the surface with non-stick cooking spray.

- From the batter mixture, scoop out $^1/_3$ cup and pour on the heated surface. Allow the pancake to spread until about 4 – 4 ½ inches in diameter and allow to cook for about 3 – 4 minutes per side.

- Repeat the above step for the remaining batter mixture.

Nutrition Facts: Calories – 164, Total Fat – 8.2g, Saturated Fat – 6.4g, Cholesterol – 22mg, Sodium – 155mg, Total Carbohydrates – 21.2g, Dietary Fiber – 2.2g, Total Sugars –

7.8g, Protein – 2g, Vitamin D – 2mcg, Calcium – 45mg, Iron – 1mg, Potassium – 92mg.

AIP-FRIENDLY GRANOLA

Cook Time: 10 minutes

Yield: 4 serves

Ingredients

- 2 cups of coconut flakes
- 1 tbsp of coconut manna
- 1 tbsp of coconut oil
- 1 pinch of salt
- ½ tsp of cinnamon
- Zest of an orange

Instructions

- Place coconut oil and coconut manna in a saucepan. Heat mix until liquid and add cinnamon. Remove from the heat source when a pourable blend is achieved.
- Prepare a mixing bowl, add coconut flakes, and pour the coconut oil mix on it and stir gently.

- Add a pinch of salt to the mix in the bowl, and then zest the orange over the mix. Stir again.
- Distribute the coconut flake mixture evenly on a cookie sheet
- Then, bake the coconut flake mixture for 15 minutes in an oven with a temperature of about 350°C. Stir occasionally to ensure an even browning of the mixture.
- Remove from the oven and allow to cool.

Nutrition Facts: Calories – 181, Total Fat – 19g, Saturated Fat – 16.8g, Cholesterol – 0mg, Sodium – 48mg, Total Carbohydrates – 7.3g, Dietary Fiber – 4.5g, Total Sugars – 2.7g, Protein – 1.6g, Calcium – 6mg, Iron – 6mg, Potassium 144mg.

AVOCADO CHICKEN SALAD

Cook Time: 30 minutes

Yield: 4 Serves

Ingredients

- 1½ pounds of chicken breasts
- 2 green onions (crushed)
- 2 tablespoons of coconut oil
- ½ bunch of Cilantro (crushed)
- 3 large Avocados
- ½ teaspoon of garlic powder
- 1 lime (juiced)
- 8 ounces of baby salad greens
- 1 tablespoon of coarse sea salt

Instructions

- Prepare a saucepan, add coconut oil, and sauté the chicken in it over medium-high heat. Cook until chicken cooks through and turns brown on the surface. Place it aside.
- Juice the lime, mince the cilantro and green onion, and then peel and chop the avocados.

- Dice the chicken (when it is cool) into ½ inch cubes.

- Then mix all the ingredients in a sizable mixing bowl, excluding the baby salad greens.

- Mash the mixture with a fork and add extra sea salt to taste. Combine well and serve over the greens.

Nutrition Facts: Calories – 644, Total Fat – 40g, Saturated Fat – 11g, Carbohydrates – 23g, Protein – 43g, Dietary Fiber – 16g, Cholesterol – 123mg, Sodium – 581mg, Sugars – 3g.

BRUSSELS SPROUT COLESLAW

Cook Time: 20 minutes

Yield: 6 serves

Ingredients

- 1 tbsp. of apple cider vinegar
- 1 small garlic clove (crushed)
- 1 tbsp. of AIP mustard (KC natural imitation mustard)
- 2 tsp of honey
- 1 red onion
- 1/3 cup of dried cherries (diced)
- 2 tsp of olive oil
- 1 pound of Brussels sprouts

Instructions

- Prepare a mixing bowl and whisk together the vinegar, mustard, honey, and crushed garlic clove. Add olive oil and stir till it's blended
- Prepare another dish and put the brussels sprout in it with the onion and cherries. Then, toss with the dressing and cover-up.
- Refrigerate for about an hour

Nutrition Facts: Calories – 123, Total Fat – 6.7g, Saturated Fat – 0.9g, Cholesterol – 0mg, Sodium – 56mg, Total Carbohydrates – 15.2g, Dietary Fiber – 3.7g, Total Sugars – 7.8g, Protein – 3.2g, Iron – 1mg, Potassium – 339mg, Calcium – 34mg.

AVOCADO KALE SALAD WITH STRAWBERRY

Cook Time: 15 minutes

Yield: 4 serves

Ingredients

- 2 bunches of Kale
- 8 oz. of strawberries (sliced)
- 1 avocado (diced)
- 1 tbsp. of pure maple syrup
- 2 tbsp. of lime juice
- Salt

Instructions

- Rinse the kale thoroughly and dry the leaves using a kitchen towel. Remember to remove the tough ribs, then chop the kale into small pieces and transfer into a bowl.
- Divide the diced avocado into two halves. Use one half to rub the kale with a pinch of salt until the kale is tender and there is a notable reduction in the size.
- Then, add the lime juice and maple syrup and toss the mixture together to be well coated.

- Put the kale salad in a dish and top with the other avocado half and the strawberries.
- Serve immediately or store in the fridge until it is ready to be served.

Nutrition Facts: Calories – 241, Carbohydrates – 20g, Protein – 6g, Total Fat – 17g, Saturated Fat – 2g, Sodium – 29mg, Sugar – 6g, Dietary Fiber – 5g, Iron 1.9mg, Vitamin C – 118.6mg, Calcium – 132mg, Potassium – 725mg, Vitamin A – 6565IU.

ZUCCHINI NOODLE

Cook Time: 20 minutes

Yield: 3 – 4 Serves

Ingredients

- 1 can of black olives (sliced)
- 2 zucchinis (medium)
- 3 pieces of cooked turkey bacon or beef strips (diced)
- ½ cup of carrots (shredded)
- ½ cup of dairy-free ranch dressing
- 2 tablespoons of fresh parsley
- 1 teaspoon of sea salt
- 1 tablespoon of coconut oil

Instructions

- Prepare a cooking pan, add oil, and apply low heat.
- Using a spiralizer, spiralize the zucchinis and cook for about 3 minutes.
- Remove the zucchini noodles and drain away from the excess water, if any.

- Place the zucchini noodles in a large bowl and add turkey bacon or beef strips, olives, and carrots to the bowl
- Stir in the ranch dressing and top with salt and parsley
- Serve chilled.

Nutrition Facts: Calories – 169, Total Fat – 10.8g, Saturated Fat – 2.5g, Cholesterol – 18mg, Sodium – 1060mg, Total Carbohydrate – 12.6g, Dietary Fiber – 15g, Total Sugars – 3.9g, Protein – 6.7g, Calcium – 37mg, Iron – 1mg, Potassium – 423mg.

WARM PORRIDGE WITH LEMON

Cook Time: 50 minutes

Yield: 4 serves

Ingredients

- 1 large head cauliflower (about 840g)
- ¾ cup of coconut (finely shredded)
- 2 tablespoons of coconut butter
- 3 cups of coconut milk
- Salt
- Zest of a lemon

Instructions

- Cut the cauliflower into florets and place them in your food processor together with the stalks.
- Pulse the cauliflower for about 10 minutes until it is the same consistency as the grains of rice.
- Then, transfer the cauliflower to a large saucepan and add the other porridge ingredients. Carefully mix.
- Apply heat to the mix and allow it to simmer, then cover up and cook for about 30 minutes until the cauliflower is tender.

- Serve porridge with berries, toasted chips, or coconut cream as desired.

Nutrition Facts: Calories – 675, Total Fat – 59.8g, Saturated Fat – 44.3g, Sodium – 129mg, Cholesterol – 0mg, Total Carbohydrate – 35.6g, Dietary Fiber – 10.6g, Total Sugars – 19.2g, Protein – 14.6g, Calcium – 75mg, Iron – 6mg, Potassium – 1163mg.

CHICKEN AND TARRAGON SAUSAGE

Cook Time: 15 minutes

Yield: 4 Serves

Ingredients

- 1 pound of ground chicken
- 1 tsp of salt
- 2 tbsp. of tarragon (finely diced)
- 4 tbsp. of coconut oil

Instructions

- Prepare a mixing bowl and in it, combine the ground chicken, diced tarragon, and salt.
- Evenly divide the mixture into 8 parts and shape each piece into a flat sausage patty.
- Prepare a saucepan, add coconut oil, and apply low heat.
- Then, fry all sides of the sausages for about 15 minutes.

Nutrition Facts: Calories – 335, Total Fat – 22.1g, Saturated Fat – 14.1g, Cholesterol – 101mg, Sodium – 679mg, Total Carbohydrate – 0.5g, Dietary Fiber – 0.1g, Total Sugars – 0g,

Protein – 33g, Calcium – 28mg, Iron – 2mg, Potassium – 303mg.

CHAPTER 6: APPETIZER, SNACKS, AND DIPS

DAIRY-FREE GINGER AND TURMERIC FRUIT DRINK

Yield: 1 serve

Cook Time: 5 minutes

Ingredients

- ½ of banana (frozen)
- 8 – 10 oz. of almond milk (unsweetened)
- 1 handful of peaches (frozen)
- 1 tsp of raw honey
- 1 tbsp. of tiger-nuts
- 1 tsp of cinnamon
- ½ teaspoon of ginger
- 1 teaspoon of turmeric

Instructions

- Combine all the ingredients in a blender and blend until the mix is smooth.

Nutrition Facts: Calories – 122, Total Fat – 2.8g, Cholesterol – 0g, Total Carbohydrate – 24.4g, Dietary Fiber – 5.5g, Sugars – 13.2g, Protein – 2.4g

AVOCADO FRIES

Yield: 24 serves

Cook Time: 25 minutes

Ingredients

- 21 strips of turkey bacon

- 3 avocados

- Ranch dressing

Instructions

- Slice the avocados each into 7 even wedges and wrap each wedge in the bacon.

- Cut turkey bacon if required and place the wedges on a baking sheet (seam side down)

- Heat up the oven to about 425°C and bake the bacon for about 15 minutes.

- Serve with dressing.

Nutrition Facts: Calories – 120, Protein – 4g, Sodium – 190mg, Fiber – 2g, Sugar – 0g, Carbohydrates – 3g, Fat – 11g, Saturated fat – 2g.

COCONUT TURMERIC BALLS

Cook Time: 10 minutes

Yield: 4 Serves

Ingredients

- 1¼ cups of shredded coconut (unsweetened)

- 1 tbsp. of turmeric powder

- ½ cup of coconut butter

- 3 tbsp. of raw honey

Instructions

- Slightly melt the raw honey and coconut butter.

- Then, stir in the shredded coconut and powder into the mix.

- Use a spoon to place the mix into ice cube trays and allow to freeze for about 2 hours.

- Allow the balls to defrost for about 10 minutes before serving

Nutrition Facts: Calories – 410, Protein – 4g, Fat – 35g, Sugar – 12g, Fiber – 9g, Carbohydrates – 23g.

RED SALSA

Cook Time: 5 minutes

Yield: 2 Serves

Ingredients

- 1/3 cup of canned beets (diced)

- 1 – 14.5 ounces of can carrots

- ½ bunch of Cilantro

- Onion (white)

- 3 tablespoons of lime juice

- ½ teaspoon of sea salt

Instructions

- Combine all the ingredients in a food processor and process carefully. A blender can also be used, but remember to pulse if running on high speed to avoid getting a liquid. It is best to process the mix on low speed to get the required salsa.

Nutrition Facts: Calories per serve – 41, Fat – 0.34g, Carbohydrate – 9.19g, Protein – 1.63g.

GARLIC KALE CHIPS

Cook Time: 5 minutes

Yield: 2 Serves

Ingredients

- 3.5 ounces of Kale

- Garlic powder

- 1 tbsp. of olive oil

- 1 tbsp. of nutritional yeast

Instructions

- Heat up the oven to about 200 °C.

- Prepare a large bowl, place the kale in it and drizzle the oil over the bowl. Make the Kale evenly coated with the drizzled oil.

- Prepare a large baking tray and place the kale evenly on it.

- Then, bake in the preheated oven for about 5 minutes.

- Remove from the oven and sprinkle garlic and yeast on the baked kale

Nutrition Facts: Calories per serve – 95, Protein – 4g, Fat, 7g, Sugar – 1g, Carbohydrate – 7g, Fiber – 3g.

SWEET POTATO SKINS (STUFFED)

Cook Time: 1 hour 30 minutes

Yield: 6 Serves

Ingredients

- 4 slices of turkey bacon (diced)

- 1/3 cup of Cilantro (diced)

- 2 Scallions (diced)

- 2 cups of mushrooms (diced)

- 1 cup of diced red onion

- ¼ tsp of fine sea salt

- ½ avocado (diced)

- 3 sweet potatoes

- 1/3 tsp of fine sea salt

- 2 tbsp. of avocado oil

- 1 pinch of salt

- 2 tsp of lemon juice

- ½ cup of coconut milk (full fat)

- 1/3 cup of diced Cilantro

(The first 7 ingredients are for the stuffing while the last 4 ingredients are for the sauce)

Instructions

- Heat the oven to about 400 ºF

- Line a broiler pan with parchment paper. Put the potatoes in the pan and bake in the oven for about 50 minutes. The potatoes should be well cooked by that time.

- Prepare a saucepan and cook the turkey bacon until brown (for about 8 minutes). Remove the turkey bacon and set aside.

- Add the mushrooms and the onion to the saucepan and cook for 12 minutes while stirring occasionally. Remove the heat source and return the turkey bacon into the saucepan. Set the stuffing aside.

- Remove the baked potatoes from the oven and allow to cool. Then, cut the potatoes in halves and scoop out the flesh using a spoon (leave about ¼ inches of the potato flesh with the skin).

- Drizzle oil and sprinkle salt on both sides of the sweet potatoes.

- Place the broiler pan back in the oven and increase the temperature to 450 °F.

- Bake the potato skins for 10 minutes on each side.

- Remove from the oven after 10 minutes and allow to cool.

- Combine the coconut milk, cilantro, lemon juice, and salt in a blender to prepare the sauce. Blend on high speed and set aside.

- Then, combine the turkey bacon, mushrooms, onions, avocado, scallions, and cilantro in a large bowl.

- Spoon the stuffing into the potato skins and top with the sauce as much as desired.

Nutrition Facts: Calories – 140, Total Fat – 8g, Saturated fat – 1g, Carbohydrate – 16g, Net Carbohydrate – 15g, Protein – 1g, Sodium – 110mg, Sugar – 2g, Fiber – 1g.

BARBEQUE BUNS

Cook Time: 1 hour

Ingredients

- 4 green plantains

- 2 tablespoons of olive oil

- 1 clove garlic (crushed)

- 1 teaspoon of sea salt

- 1 tablespoon of beef gelatin

- 1 tablespoon of cold water

- 2 tablespoons of hot water

- 1 tablespoon of olive oil

- Coarse sea salt

Instructions

- Heat up the oven to about 435 °C.

- Peel 2 of the 4 green plantains and chop them into chunks.

- Put the pieces in a clean pot and cover with water.

- Apply heat and boil until tender.

- Peel the remaining 2 plantains and grate them. Put the shredded plantains into a large bowl and set aside

- Drain the water away from the boiled plantain chunks and add the pieces to the food processor.

- Add the two tablespoons of olive oil, minced garlic, salt, and blend them until a ball of smoothly pureed plantain is achieved.

- Then, add the ball of plantain to the large mixing bowl containing the shredded plantains

- Inside another bowl, combine the beef gelatin with 1 tablespoon of cold water and continuously stir until uniform. Add 2 tablespoons of hot water and stir until the gelatin is dissolved.

- Add the gelatin mix to the plantain mix and combine using a mixer until they are smoothly blended.

- Transfer the dough to a piece of parchment paper and cover with another piece of parchment paper (you can also use a silicone baking mat).

- Roll or mat the dough until the thickness is about ½ inch.

- Continue to roll and cut out circles until there is no more dough.

- Fold up the sides and roll them until entirely shaped like balls.

- Drizzle olive oil on the buns and sprinkle the coarse sea salt on them — Bake for 20 – 25 minutes.

Nutrition Facts: Calories – 440, Fat – 31g, Protein – 13g, Cholesterol – 62mg, Sodium – 214mg, Saturated Fat – 10g, Sugar – 15g, Carbohydrate – 31g.

CHICKEN AVOCADO

Cook Time: 20 minutes

Yield: 2 – 4 Serves

Ingredients

- 3 cloves garlic, minced

- 1 tbsp. of coconut oil

- ½ tsp of dried oregano leaves

- ¼ cup of lemon juice

- ¼ cup of orange juice

- ½ pound of shredded chicken

- ½ onion (small)

- 2 avocados

- 1 mango

- ¼ cup of fresh cilantro leaves (diced)

- Pinch salt

- 1 tbsp. of lime juice

Instructions

- Add ½ tablespoon of coconut oil and crushed garlic to a saucepan. Cook until garlic softens and gives a pleasant smell, that should take about a minute.

- Add the orange juice, oregano leaves, and the lemon juice to the saucepan to make mojo sauce.

- Apply low heat and bring the juice to a simmer, then cook for a few minutes.

- Transfer the mojo sauce into a jar and set aside.

- Pour the remaining coconut oil into the saucepan and apply medium heat. Add the shredded chicken and cook.

- Finely slice the onion and add it to the saucepan. Add four tablespoons of the mojo sauce and toss to coat. Reduce heat and cover-up — Cook for about 8 minutes.

- Then, pour the remaining mojo sauce into the saucepan and cover-up. Remove from heat and allow to cool.

- Ensure the avocados are cut in half and the pit removed. Cut a small slice from the rounded end of the avocado halves and discard to prevent instability on the plate.

- Divide the mojo chicken evenly between the avocado halves.

- Whisk together the mango, cilantro, lime juice, and salt in a bowl. Spoon the mango mix over the mojo chicken and serve.

Nutrition Facts: Calories – 391, Total Fat – 25.3g, Saturated Fat – 7.8g, Cholesterol – 44mg, Sodium – 87mg, Total Carbohydrate – 25.6g, Dietary Fiber – 8.6g, Total Sugars – 14.3g, Protein – 19.6g, Calcium – 41mg, Iron – 2mg, Potassium 825mg.

CHICKEN TENDERS

Cook Time: 45 minutes

Yield: 4 Serves

Ingredients

- 2 cups of plantain chips with sea salt

- 1 pound of organic chicken tenders

- 2 tsp of onion powder

- 1 tsp of garlic powder

- 2 tbsp. of cassava flour

- 1 cup of coconut milk

- 3 tbsp. of apple cider vinegar

- 1 tsp of sea salt

Instructions

- Heat the oven to about 375 ºC, line the roasting pan with foil, and place the roasting rack on top.

- Process the plantain chips, cassava flour, onion powder, garlic powder, and sea salt in a food processor until a relatively fine crumb is achieved and transfer into a bowl.

- Whisk the coconut milk and vinegar together in another mixing bowl.

- Then, dip each chicken tenders in the coconut milk mix and then, in the crumb and place them on the roasting rack. (Allow the chicken tenders to drain off a little after dipping in the first liquid; i.e., coconut milk mix before dipping into the crumb).

- Bake the tenders for about 30 minutes or until the desired color is achieved.

Nutrition Facts: Calories – 112, Total Fat – 6.2g, Saturated Fat – 1.1g, Dietary Fiber – 0.3g, Sugar – 0.1g, Total Carbohydrate – 7.1g, Cholesterol – 17mg, Sodium – 296mg, Potassium – 120mg, Protein – 7g.

APPLE SALSA

Cook Time: 15 minutes

Yield: 2 Serves

Ingredients

- 1 cup of Apples (peeled and diced)

- ½ cup of cucumbers (peeled and diced)

- Salt

- ¼ cup of shallots (diced)

- ¼ cup of cilantro (diced)

- 2 tablespoons of apple vinegar

Instructions

- Prepare a mixing bowl and in it, combine all the ingredients.

- Stir well to mix and serve.

Nutrition Facts: Calories – 41, Carbohydrate – 10g, Sugar – 7g, Fiber – 2g, Fat – 1g, Protein – 1g, Saturated Fat – 1g, Sodium – 3mg, Potassium – 112mg.

CAULIFLOWER DIP

Cook Time: 40 minutes

Yield: 2 Serves

Ingredients

- ½ head of cauliflower

- 3 tablespoons of olive oil

- 2 tablespoons of lemon juice

- 3 cloves of unpeeled garlic

- Sea salt

Instructions

- Heat your oven to about 200 ºC.

- Break the cauliflower into florets. Place the florets in a mixing bowl, add 2 tablespoons of olive oil and whisk together.

- Spread the florets out on a greased baking tray. Put the unpeeled cloves in an air-tight foil parcel and put together with the florets on the baking tray.

- Allow roasting in the pre-heated oven for about 30 minutes. (Toss the florets after 15 minutes for evenness).

- After roasting, transfer the soft roasted florets into a small food processor.

- Gently open the parcel containing the garlic cloves and squeeze the roasted flesh from the skins into the food processor. Add lemon juice and olive oil, then blitz the mix until a smooth puree is achieved. Add salt to taste and serve

- It may be served with radishes and cucumber sticks or any preferred vegetable.

Nutrition Facts: Calories per serve – 225, Sugar – 5g, Protein – 3g, Fat – 21g, Carbohydrates – 10g, Fiber – 4g.

AVOCADO DIP

Cook Time: 20 minutes

Yield: 6 – 8 Serves

Ingredients

- 2 carrots

- ¼ cup of onion (brown)

- 10 sprigs of Parsley

- 1 garlic clove

- 1 whole oregano

- 1 tbsp. of olive oil

- 2 tbsp. of apple cider vinegar

- 2 tbsp. of nutritional yeast

- ¼ tsp of sea salt

- 2 avocados

Instructions

- In a mixing bowl, combine the vinegar, olive oil, oregano, nutritional yeast, and salt.

- Then, mince the garlic clove and add to the mixing bowl.

- Chop the onion, carrots, and avocado and add to the mixing bowl.

- Mince the parsley and add to the mix.

- Then stir gently to allow the ingredients mix well.

- Allow to sit for a few minutes before serving.

Nutrition Facts: Calories – 235, Total Fat – 14.03g, Saturated Fat – 1.45g, Cholesterol – 0mg, Sodium – 116mg, Potassium – 352.75mg, Dietary Fiber – 5.38g, Carbohydrates – 11.12g, Sugar – 2.12g, Protein – 2.12g, Calcium – 14.25mg, Vitamin C – 31.06mg, Iron – 1.88mg.

AVOCADO CRACK DIP

Cook Time: 5 minutes

Yield: 2 Serves

Ingredients

- 1 pint of zucchini (diced)

- ¼ cup of onion (diced)

- ½ teaspoon of oregano

- 1 bunch of parsley (finely diced)

- 1 tablespoon of olive oil

- 1 crushed garlic clove

- 2 tablespoons of red wine vinegar

- 2 tablespoons of nutritional yeast

- 2 large avocados

- Salt to taste

Instruction:

- Prepare a mixing bowl and combine all ingredients in it except for the avocados.

- Continuously stir to combine the mix. Cover up and refrigerate for several hours or better still, overnight.

- After refrigerating, chop the avocados into small chunks and add them to the bowl. Stir well before serving.

- Best served with sweet potato chips.

Nutrition Facts: Calories – 621, Total Fat – 50.1g, Saturated Fat 15.5g, Cholesterol – 50mg, Sodium – 730mg, Total Carbohydrate – 35.7g, Dietary Fiber – 19.9g, Total Sugars – 15.2g, Protein – 16.9g, Calcium – 348mg, Iron – 2mg, Potassium – 1601mg.

BLACKBERRY JAM

Cook Time: 15 minutes

Yield: 2 cups

Ingredients

- 2 cups of blackberries

- 2 cups of coconut sugar

- 2 tbsp. of lemon juice

Instructions

- Prepare a large saucepan, preferably an enamel saucepan. Put the berries in it and boil over high heat. Mash the berries as they boil, add the lemon juice and stir while still mashing.

- Add the coconut sugar and bring the mix back to a boil. Stir continuously and allow to cook for about 5 minutes until the mix thickens a little.

- Then, remove the heat source and test if it's done. The mix will coat the back of a spoon if it is done. A candy thermometer showing 220 °F also means the mix is ready. If otherwise, apply heat again for a few minutes but avoid letting the mixture get too thick while being heated.

- Transfer the jam to a jar when it is done and allow it to cool to room temperature (that should take about a couple hours).

- After cooling, cover the jar with a well-fitted lid and refrigerate.

Nutrition Facts: Calories per tablespoon serve – 50, Total Fat – 0g, Carbohydrates – 13g, Sugar – 12g

CHAPTER 7: SALAD, SOUP, AND SIDES

CHICKEN NOODLE SOUP USING INSTANT POT

Cook Time: 30 minutes

Yield: 8 Serves

Ingredients

- 2 tablespoons of coconut butter

- 1 onion (diced)

- 1 tablespoon of fresh parsley (diced)

- 2 medium-sized carrots (diced)

- 1 teaspoon of salt

- 2 stalks of celery (diced)

- 4 cups of chicken broth

- 1 teaspoon of dry thyme

- 1 tablespoon of fresh oregano (diced)

- 2 pounds of chicken with skin and bones

- 4 cups of water

- 2 cups of egg noodles (uncooked)

Instructions

- Prepare your instant pot; turn it to the sauté setting.

- Add the coconut butter to the pot and cook until it melts. Add onion, carrots, and celery to the pot and sauté for about 3 minutes, until it becomes translucent

- Add salt to taste. Stir in thyme, parsley, oregano, and the chicken broth. Pour 4 cups of water into the pot and add the chicken pieces.

- Then, close the lid and set the pot to the soup setting. Also, set the timer to 7 minutes.

- When the timer is done, allow the natural release cycle to be complete before carefully unlocking the lid.

- When the lid is unlocked, remove the chicken pieces from the soup and shred using two forks.

- Then, add the egg noodles to the soup and set the instant pot back to the sauté setting. Cook the noodles while the pot is uncovered for about 6 – 7 minutes, after which you should turn off the instant pot using the 'cancel' button.

- Then, add the shredded chicken back to the pot and taste to know if seasoning needs adjustment before serving.

Nutrition Facts: Calories – 374, Total Fat – 21g, Carbohydrate – 18g, Saturated Fat – 7g, Protein – 26g, Cholesterol – 107mg, Sodium – 435mg, Potassium – 469mg, Iron – 2mg, Sugar – 2g, Calcium – 50mg, Fiber – 1g, Vitamin C – 5.2mg, Vitamin A – 2900IU.

BUTTERNUT SQUASH SOUP USING INSTANT POT

Cook Time: 30 minutes

Yield: 4 – 6 Serves

Ingredients

- 1 organic butternut squash (diced)

- 1 onion (diced)

- 2 pints of organic chicken broth

- 1 teaspoon of ground cinnamon

- ½ teaspoon of salt

- 2 tablespoons of avocado oil

Instructions

- Prepare your instant pot and turn it to the sauté setting.

- Add the avocado oil to the pot and sauté the diced onion in it.

- Add the cinnamon and salt when translucent.

100

- Add the peeled and diced butternut squash to the instant pot and pour in the chicken broth.

- Turn off the instant pot. Turn it on again to manual for about 2 minutes and quickly release the pressure.

- Then, pour the mixture into a food processor and puree.

Nutrition Facts: Calories per serve – 82, Protein – 1.8g, Fat – 0.18g, Potassium – 582mg, Dietary Fiber – 6.6g, Sugar – 4g, Carbohydrate – 21.5g, Calcium – 84mg, Phosphorus – 55mg, Magnesium – 59mg, Vitamin C – 31mg.

GREEN SALAD WITH ITALIAN DRESSING

Cook Time: 15 minutes

Yield: 8 Serves

Ingredients

- 1 crushed garlic clove

- 3 tbsp. of lemon juice

- ¼ cup of olive oil

- 4 oz. of mesclun

- 1 cucumber

- 16 oz. of zucchini (chopped)

- 1 tbsp. of parsley (diced)

- 1 tsp of dried oregano

- 1 tsp of Italian seasoning

- Salt

- 1 head of Boston lettuce (torn)

Instructions

- Prepare a mixing bowl and combine the olive oil, lemon juice, oregano, parsley, garlic clove, and Italian seasoning until it blends. Add salt to taste.

- Toss the remaining ingredients together in a large bowl with the dressing and serve.

Nutrition Facts: Calories per serve – 80, Carbohydrate – 12g, Fat – 2g, Protein – 2g, Dietary Fiber – 1g, Sugar – 3g, Sodium – 730mg.

FENNEL CURRY AND SWEET POTATO

Cook Time: 50 minutes

Yield: 4 Serves

Ingredients

- 4 cups of sweet potato (peeled and cubed)

- 3 tsp of olive oil

- 1 cup of fennel (diced)

- 1 cup of red onion (diced)

- 2 tbsp. of fresh mint (diced)

- ¼ cup of fresh cilantro

- 2 tsp of coconut oil

- 2 tbsp. of curry powder

- ¼ tsp of sea salt

- 1 cup of cooked chickpeas

- ½ juice of a lemon

Instructions

- Heat up the oven to about 400 °F.

- Get a baking sheet, sprinkle with olive oil, and lay-out the peeled and cubed sweet potatoes on it.

- Allow to roast in the preheated oven for about 40 minutes until the potatoes are soft (not mushy); then, remove and set aside.

- In a pan, add coconut oil, onion, curry powder, fennel, and salt. Sauté over medium heat for about 7 minutes.

- In a bowl, combine the fennel mix with the remaining ingredients and the roasted potatoes.

- Stir the mix to be well coated and serve.

Nutrition Facts: Calories – 444, Total Fat – 9.7g, Saturated Fat – 2.9g, Cholesterol – 0mg, Sodium – 218mg, Total Carbohydrate – 78.2g, Dietary Fiber – 18g, Total Sugars – 19.8g, Protein – 14.8g, Calcium – 99mg, Iron – 12mg, Potassium – 1594mg.

LIME CILANTRO CAULIFLOWER

Cook Time: 20 minutes

Yield: 6 Serves

Ingredients

- 3 cups of cauliflower rice

- 1 tbsp. of olive oil

- ½ cup of diced onion (white)

- 1 tbsp. of lime juice

- 1 tsp of garlic clove

- 2 tbsp. of vegetable stock

- ½ cup of freshly diced cilantro

- Salt

- Zest from halved lime

Instructions

- Prepare a large saucepan, pour the olive oil in it, and apply medium heat.

- Sauté the onions for 5 minutes until they become translucent.

- Add the garlic clove and cook while stirring. Add the cauliflower rice to the saucepan and stir the mix to combine well.

- Divide the cilantro into two and add one part to the saucepan together with the vegetable stock, salt, lime zest, and then stir. Increase the heat and allow to cook for about a minute. Then reduce the heat and add the lime juice.

- Add salt to taste and stir in the remaining cilantro.

- Cauliflower cilantro rice is ready, serve warm.

Nutrition Facts: Calories per serve – 48, Protein – 1g, Sodium – 239mg, Carbohydrate – 5g, Fiber – 1g, Sugar – 2g.

ROASTED VEGETABLE WITH DRESSING

Cook Time: 1 hour

Yield: 4 Serves

Ingredients

- ½ large cauliflower

- 3 tablespoons of coconut oil (melted)

- 8 peeled baby brown shallots

- Zest of a large lemon

- ½ a bunch of black kale

- 1 halved delicata squash

- Sea salt

- 1 bunch of radishes

- 8 asparagus stalks (diced without the woody part)

- 4 tablespoons of olive oil

- 3 tablespoons of lemon juice

- 1 tablespoon of raw vinegar (apple cider)

- 1 tablespoon of raw honey

- Sea salt

(The last five ingredients are for the dressing)

Instructions

- Heat up the oven to about 400 ºF.

- Prepare a roasting pan and divide the coconut oil. Add 2 tablespoons of the coconut oil to the pan together with the squash and shallots. Turn the veggies over in the coconut oil until they are well coated (you may use your hand to achieve a better coating).

- Add the zest and whisk the vegetables again, and then sprinkle sea salt over the veggies and put the pan in the preheated oven for about 20 minutes.

- Afterward, add the radishes, kale, asparagus, and whisk together again. Put the pan back in the oven for another 20 minutes.

- Cut the cauliflower into florets and process them in a food processor with the S-shaped blade and then pulse the florets until the size of large grains of rice is achieved.

- Prepare a saucepan and heat the remaining coconut oil in it. Add the cauliflower rice and allow it to cook for four minutes with medium heat until the rice becomes tender.

- Prepare the dressing by whisking the ingredients together in a mixing bowl.

- Transfer the cauliflower to a serving platter, add the roasted veggies and the dressing. Carefully mix and serve.

Nutrition Facts: Calories – 332, Total Fat – 24.4g, Saturated Fat – 10.9g, Sodium – 269mg, Cholesterol – 0mg, Total Carbohydrate – 28.5g, Dietary Fiber – 3g, Total Sugars – 16.9g, Protein – 4.5g, Calcium – 29mg, Iron – 1mg, Potassium – 358mg.

STEAK SALAD WITH TARRAGON DRESSING

Cook Time: 15 minutes

Yield: 4 Serves

Ingredients

- 1¼ pounds of well-salted grass-fed steaks

- 1 tablespoon of fat

- 4½ cups of green

- 4 ounces of mushrooms (sliced)

- 1 handful of diced parsley

- 3 tablespoons of balsamic vinegar

- 2 tablespoons of crushed tarragon

- ½ cup of organic olive oil

- ½ teaspoon of salt

- ¼ teaspoon of garlic powder

The last 5 ingredients are for the Tarragon Dressing

Instructions

- Prepare a jar and add garlic powder, olive oil, tarragon, and salt to it - for the dressing. Cover up the jar, shake well and set aside.

- Get the fat of your choice and heat in a grill pan over medium heat. Cook the steaks until it is as desired, flipping the steaks once when cooking.

- Then, transfer to a board and allow to sit for some time.

- You may use a combination of lettuce, arugula, and spinach for the greens. Share the greens and the sliced mushrooms between the plates. Slice the steaks into strips and put them on the salads.

- Shake the tarragon dressing again and apply as desired. Garnish with parsley before serving.

Nutrition Facts: Calories – 337, Total Fat – 30.4g, Saturated Fat – 5.7g, Cholesterol – 8mg, Sodium – 366mg, Total Carbohydrate – 12.1g, Dietary Fiber – 4.1g, Total Sugars – 4.7g, Protein 6.9g, Calcium – 30mg, Iron – 2mg, Potassium – 306mg, Vitamin D – 102mcg.

GREEN SALAD WITH DRESSING

Cook Time: 10 minutes

Yield: 8 Serves

Ingredients

- 2 stalks of finely sliced celery

- About 12 cups of salad greens

- 1 ½ cucumber (sliced)

- 2 cups of sunflower sprouts

- 2 tbsp. of fish sauce

- ¼ cup of fresh lime juice

- 1 garlic clove (crushed)

- ½ tsp of honey

- 2 tbsp. of diced cilantro (fresh)

- 1 tbsp. of diced mint (fresh)

The last six ingredients are for the dressing

Instructions

- Prepare a bowl and whisk together the salad ingredients – greens, celery, cucumbers, and the sunflower sprouts.

- In another bowl, combine the ingredients for the dressing together and blend using a blender for about 20 seconds. If the cilantro and mint are finely diced, you can alternatively choose to mix the ingredients by hand merely.

- Serve salad with the dressing.

Nutrition Facts: Calories – 106, Total Fat – 1.1g, Saturated Fat – 0g, Cholesterol – 0mg, Sodium – 413mg, Total Carbohydrate – 19.9g, Dietary Fiber – 8.8g, Total Sugars – 9.7g, Protein – 5.3g, Calcium – 178mg, Iron – 3mg, Potassium 118mg.

LEMON TUNA SALAD

Cook Time: 10 minutes

Yield: 1 Serve

Ingredients

- ½ small avocado (diced)

- 1 can of tuna (about 6 ounces)

- 1/3 small cucumber (diced)

- 1 tsp of lemon juice

- Salt

- Salad greens (if desired)

- 1 tbsp. of olive oil

Instructions

- Combine the cucumber, avocado, and lemon juice in a medium bowl. Flake the tuna and add to the cucumber mix. Add salt to taste

- If desired, prepare the salad greens adding olive oil and lemon juice to taste.

115

- Serve the salad greens and place the tuna salad on top.

Nutrition Facts: Calories – 480, Sugar – 2g, Fat – 40g, Carbohydrate – 11g, Fiber – 8g, Protein – 45g.

NOTATO SALAD WITH DRESSING

Cook Time: 2 hours 35 minutes

Yield: 8 Serves

Ingredients

- 12 cups of a combination of different vegetables (about 3 – 4 types) sliced into ½ inch pieces

- 3 stalks of celery (finely diced)

- ½ cup of red onion (finely diced)

- 3 tbsp. of palm shortening for the dressing

- 1 tsp of salt

- ¼ tsp of turmeric

- 1 tbsp. of dried dill

- 2 tbsp. of olive oil

- ¼ tsp of wasabi powder

- 1 tbsp. of fresh lemon juice

- ½ cup of plain coconut milk

The last 8 ingredients are for the dressing

Instructions

- Using a steamer basket, steam the vegetables individually until vegetables are soft but not mushy.

- After steaming, transfer into a bowl and refrigerate for about 2 hours.

- Add celery and onion after refrigerating.

- Whisk together the ingredients for the dressing until the mix becomes light and fluffy (use a hand mixer for about 4 – 5 minutes).

- Then, fold the dressing into the root vegetable mixture and serve.

Nutrition Facts: Calories – 211, Total Fat – 9.8g, Saturated Fat – 4.5g, Cholesterol – 0mg, Sodium – 662mg, Total Carbohydrate – 25.3g, Dietary Fiber – 8.1g, Total Sugars – 7.3g, Protein – 6.6g.

SARDINE SALAD

Cook Time: 5 minutes

Yield: 1 Serve

Ingredients

- 5 ounces of sardine in olive oil (1 can)

- Salt

- 1 tbsp. of olive oil

- 1/10 pound of beef deli meat (diced)

- 1 tbsp. of lemon juice

- ¼ pound of salad greens

Instructions

- Toss the salad greens with olive oil and lemon juice to prepare the salad. Add the deli meat and toss again.

- Drain the sardines and top the salad with it.

- Drizzle salt over the sardine salad to taste.

Nutrition Facts: Calories – 400, Protein – 30g, Fiber – 1g, Carbohydrates – 2g, Fat – 34g, Sugar – 0g.

MELON SALAD

Cook Time: 5 minutes

Yield: 2 Serves

Ingredients

- ½ small cucumber

- ½ small melon

- 2 handfuls of salad leaves

- Sea salt

- 2 tbsp. of olive oil

- 1 tbsp. of fresh ginger (diced)

- 2 tsp of fresh lemon juice

Instructions

- Combine everything in a dish bowl and toss together to mix. Your salad is ready.

Nutrition Facts: Calories – 172, Fat – 14g, Protein – 3g, Cholesterol – 0g, Fiber – 3g, Sugar – 9g, Carbohydrate – 12g.

SEAWEED SALAD

Cook Time: 15 minutes

Yield: 8 Serves

Ingredients

- 2 cups of finely sliced cucumber

- 2 cups of finely sliced daikon radish (or turnip)

- 2 tsp of honey

- ¼ cup of fresh lemon juice

- 2 tbsp. of coconut water vinegar

- 4 tsp of fish sauce

- 2 green onions (finely diced)

- 2 oz. of dried seaweed

- 1 tsp of fresh ginger juice

Instructions

- Place the ginger juice, the coconut vinegar, fish sauce, honey, and lemon juice in a bowl and mix.

- Soak the seaweed in cold water for about five minutes or soak until it doesn't taste tough again.

- Rinse and drain. Then combine the seaweed, radish, cucumber, and the dressing (remember to peel the cucumber if the skin is tough). Garnish with onions and serve.

Nutrition Facts: Calories – 23, Total Fat – 0.1g, Saturated Fat – 0.1g, Cholesterol – 0mg, Sodium – 358mg, Total Carbohydrate – 7.3g, Dietary Fiber – 0.8g, Total Sugars – 4.5g, Protein – 1.2g.

SASHIMI SALAD

Cook Time: 15 minutes

Yield: 2 Serves

Ingredients

- 1 Ataulfo mango

- 2 tbsp. of olive oil

- 1 tsp of balsamic vinegar

- 2 handfuls of baby kale leaves

- ½ pound of salmon sashimi

- ½ tbsp. of raw honey

- 2 tbsp. of coconut aminos

Instructions

- Peel the mango and slice it. Also, slice the sashimi into about 12 slices.

- Combine the honey, coconut aminos, vinegar, and oil in a bowl for the salad dressing.

- Toss the salad dressing with the kale leaves and divide into two dish bowls

- Top each bowl with the sliced mango and sashimi, and serve.

Nutrition Facts: Calories – 486, Total Fat – 23.4g, Saturated Fat – 3.5g, Cholesterol – 0mg, Total Carbohydrate – 57.8g, Sodium – 1661mg, Dietary Fiber – 8.2g, Total Sugars – 25.6g, Protein – 15.6g.

BAMBOO SALAD

Cook Time: 5 minutes

Yield: 2 Serves

Ingredients

- 1 can (about 8 ounces) of sliced bamboo shoots

- 1 tbsp. of olive oil

- 2 tbsp. of finely diced cilantro

- Salt

Instructions

- Drain the bamboo shoots and toss the shoots together with the oil and cilantro.

- Add salt to taste. Toss together and serve.

Nutrition Facts: Calories – 240, Total Fat – 7g, Saturated Fat – 1g, Cholesterol – 0mg, Sodium – 98mg, Total Carbohydrate – 32g, Dietary Fiber – 12g, Total Sugars – 0g, Protein – 12g

CHAPTER 8: VEGETABLE RECIPES

VEGETABLE SCRAMBLE

Cook Time: 30 minutes

Yield: 3 Serves

Ingredients

- 24 oz. of red cabbage (diced)

- 24 oz. of butternut squash (diced)

- 1 tsp of sea salt

- 2 tbsp. of coconut oil

- ½ cup of green onion (diced)

Instructions

- Prepare a large frying pan or skillet, apply medium heat, and melt the coconut oil.

- Add butternut squash, salt, and cabbage to the pan and then simmer for about 15 minutes while you stir occasionally.

- Ensure salt is adequate for the taste and garnish with the green onions before serving.

Nutrition Facts: Calories – 172, Total Fat – 9.3g, Saturated Fat – 7.9g, Cholesterol – 0mg, Sodium – 649mg, Total Carbohydrate – 23.1g, Dietary Fiber – 5.9g, Total Sugars – 6.7g, Protein – 2.3g.

BABY ARTICHOKES

Cook Time: 40 minutes

Yield: 4 Serves

Ingredients

- 5 pounds of baby artichokes

- 4 slices of turkey bacon

- 1 lemon

- 1 cup of water

Instructions

- Prepare a skillet, apply medium heat, and cook the turkey bacon until crispy. Turn the bacon as required until they are tender – that that should take about 15 minutes. After cooking, set the bacon aside, leaving the fat in the skillet.

- Prepare the artichoke while cooking the turkey bacon, get a bowl, and pour the water and the juiced lemon in it. Set aside the bowl.

- Then, take away most of the outer leaves of the artichokes, slash the top part, and cut it into half. Place the halves in the bowl containing water and lemon juice (this will prevent color change before cooking the artichoke).

- Apply medium-high heat to the skillet again and add the artichokes. Allow to sauté for about ten minutes and stir until it is well cooked, and the edges turn brown.

- Chop the turkey bacon into bits and serve the artichokes with the bacon on top.

Nutrition Facts: Calories – 329, Total Fat – 6.1g, Saturated Fat – 2g, Cholesterol – 15mg, Sodium – 1001mg, Total Carbohydrate – 62.7g, Dietary Fiber – 31g, Total Sugars – 10.7g, Protein – 24.5g.

ROASTED LEEK GREENS

Cook Time: 30 minutes

Yield: 2 Serves

Ingredients

- 2 cups of leek greens

- 1 tablespoon of avocado oil

- ½ teaspoon of sea salt

Instructions

- Heat up the oven to about 425 ºC. Then chop the leek greens stalk into ½ inch rounds.

- Get a salad spinner and place the diced leeks in it, rinse with water and spin dry.

- Then, transfer the leek greens into a baking dish, toss with the avocado oil and sprinkle the sea salt on it.

- When hot, put the leeks in the pre-heated oven and cook for about 20 minutes until it turns brown and becomes crispy.

Nutrition Facts: Calories – 59, Total Fat – 0.9g, Saturated Fat – 0.2g, Cholesterol – 0mg, Sodium – 483mg, Total Carbohydrate – 12.4g, Dietary Fiber – 2.3g, Total Sugars – 3g, Protein – 1.1g.

KIMCHI (ALL VEGETABLES)

Cook Time: 3 hours

Yield: 3 Serves

Ingredients

- 2 bunches of scallions (diced)

- 6 radishes

- 2 Chinese cabbages

- 1 tablespoon of ginger

- 1 ½ cups of sea salt

- 1 tablespoon of coconut aminos

- 1 apple

- 1 pear (Asian)

- 2 carrots

- 1 onion

- 2 tablespoons of crushed garlic

Instructions

- Rinse the cabbages and chop them into small pieces. Place the cabbages in a large bowl and sprinkle the sea salt over it.

- Allow the well-salted cabbages to sit in the bowl for about 2 hours until shrinkage occurs.

- Process ginger, garlic, onion, carrots, radishes, apple, and pear in a food processor to form a paste.

- Rinse the salt off the wilted cabbages and drain well. Place the cabbages back into the bowl and add in the marinade and diced scallions. Toss the mix together.

- Pack the mix into kimchi jars, ensuring there is enough headspace. Then store in a dark and cool place for days (depending on your desired level of fermentation) to allow the kimchi ferment.

- Refrigerate the kimchi when the desired level of fermentation is achieved.

Nutrition Facts: Calories – 155, Total Fat – 0.6g, Saturated Fat – 0.1g, Cholesterol – 0mg, Sodium – 44994mg, Total

Carbohydrate – 37.7g, Dietary Fiber – 8.6g, Total Sugars – 18.8g, Protein – 3.9g.

CREAMY SPINACH

Cook Time: 1 hour

Yield: 6 Serves

Ingredients

- 4 garlic cloves

- 2 onions (roughly diced)

- 2 cups of chicken broth (divided)

- ¼ cup of olive oil

- ¼ teaspoon of ground turmeric

- ¼ teaspoon of ground cloves

- Salt

- 16 oz. of frozen spinach (diced)

Instructions

- Puree the onion and the garlic cloves using a food processor. Then, prepare a large saucepot and apply medium heat.

- Pour the onion-garlic mix in the pot and cook for about 5 minutes, stirring occasionally.

- Add olive oil, turmeric, ground cloves, and the chicken broth to the pot and toss together to mix well. Cook with the pot uncovered for about 14 minutes, occasionally stirring until there's a reduction in the liquid.

- Then, add the spinach to the pot and toss to combine well. Cook for another 25 minutes adding the remaining broth to ensure a creamy mix.

- With the liquid in the pot, cook the mix for another 10 minutes, and add salt to taste. Serve.

Nutrition Facts: Calories – 109, Protein – 3g, Carbohydrate – 4g, Fat – 10g, Iron – 2mg, Sugar – 1g, Potassium – 332mg, Saturated Fat – 1g, Sodium – 343mg, Fiber – 2g, Calcium – 106mg, Vitamin C – 10mg.

MUSHROOM TURNIP GREENS WITH ALMONDS

Cook Time: 25 minutes

Yield: 6 Serves

Ingredients

- ½ cup of raw almonds

- 1 turnip greens

- 1 teaspoon of ginger (finely grated)

- 1 pound of sliced mushrooms

- 2 garlic cloves

- 2 tablespoons of coconut oil

- ¼ cup of orange juice

- 1 tablespoon of coconut aminos

- 2 teaspoons of arrowroot flour

Instructions

- Rinse the turnip greens thoroughly and combine them with the mushrooms but first slice the stems of the greens and chop the greens into small pieces. Set aside.

- Prepare a skillet and apply medium heat. Add coconut oil, garlic, and ginger for a couple of minutes and then add the mushrooms and green turnip stems.

- Cook the mix in a skillet until sticky while frequently stirring. Stir in the orange juice and continue cooking until the stems are beginning to soften.

- Add the remaining turnip leaves and the almonds and cook until fully wilted

- Add the coconut aminos and drizzle the arrowroot powder on it (as the powder thickens the remaining juices at the bottom of the skillet), frequently stir for about 4 minutes and serve.

Nutrition Facts: Calories – 142, Total Fat – 9g, Saturated Fat – 4.3g, Cholesterol – 0mg, Sodium – 20mg, Total Carbohydrate – 13.4g, Dietary Fiber – 2.9g, Total Sugars – 6.7g, Protein – 5g.

KABOCHA SQUASH WEDGES (ROASTED)

Cook Time: 45 minutes

Yield: 4 Serves

Ingredients

- 1 medium kabocha squash

- Ground ginger

- Kosher salt

- 1 tbsp. of olive oil or avocado oil.

Instructions

- Heat up the oven to about 400 ºF.

- Rinse the kabocha squash thoroughly, dry it, and peel using a vegetable peeler.

- Cut off the squash at both ends and scoop out the seeds. Then, cut the squash into thin wedges.

- With the fat of your choice, toss the squash and sprinkle salt and ginger on the squash wedges.

- Place the squash in a layer on a foil and put it in the preheated oven.

- Allow the squash to roast for about 30 minutes, ensuring to flip over after 15 minutes.

- Serve and enjoy the soft and fluffy wedges.

Nutrition Facts: Calories – 58, Total Fat – 3.6g, Saturated Fat – 0.5g, Cholesterol – 0mg, Sodium – 39mg, Total Carbohydrate – 6.2g, Dietary Fiber – 1.6g, Total Sugars – 4.5g, Protein – 0.9g.

DAIKON CONFIT HASH

Cook Time: 1 hour

Yield: 2 Serves

Ingredients

- 1 daikon radish (medium)

- 1 tsp of Himalayan salt

- About 2 cups of duck fat

- Few sprigs of crushed parsley

Instructions

- Cut the daikon radish into cubes.

- Place a pan over low heat, add the duck fat and daikon radish and allow the fat to melt slowly.

- Cook the radish gently in the fat for about 25 minutes while stirring occasionally.

- Remove heat source and sieve out the fat into a jar. Allow the sieved fat to cool and then refrigerate.

- Place the cooked daikon and the duck fat left into the pan, apply medium-high heat. Add the salt (use regular salt if you don't have Himalayan salt) and fry until the daikon turns brown.

- Garnish with crushed parsley and serve.

Nutrition Facts: Calories – 1820, Total Fat – 204.8g, Saturated Fat – 68.1g, Cholesterol – 205mg, Sodium – 306mg, Total Carbohydrate – 2.3g, Dietary Fiber – 1.2g, Total Sugars – 0.7g, Protein – 1.1g.

LIME AND BERRIES JICAMA

Cook Time: 5 minutes

Yield: 2 Serves

Ingredients

- ½ organic Jicama

- 1 lime

- ½ cup of berry mix

Instructions

- Peel the Jicama and slice into sticks.

- Ensure the organic lime is zested and juiced.

- Toss together the Jicama sticks, berry mix, and the lime in a sizable bowl.

- Serve chilled.

Nutrition Facts: Calories – 108, Total Fat – 1.1g, Saturated Fat – 0g, Cholesterol – 0mg, Sodium – 30mg, Total Carbohydrate – 24.6g, Dietary Fiber – 9.3g, Total Sugars – 7g, Protein – 1.9g.

CARROT CILANTRO MASH

Cook Time: 25 minutes

Yield: 4 Serves

Ingredients

- 2 pounds of Carrots

- ½ cup of Cilantro (roughly diced)

- 3 tablespoons of olive oil (extra virgin)

- 1 teaspoon of salt

- Pinch mace

Instructions

- Rinse carrots thoroughly and cut into ½ inch rounds.

- Place the carrots into a sizable pan with little water or, better still, place them in a steamer.

- Cover up and bring to a simmer, then cook until the carrot is tender (that should take about 15 minutes).

- Drain off the carrots and transfer them into a food processor with the S-shaped blade. Add the

145

remaining ingredients and blend until the mix is smooth.

- Serve immediately.

Nutrition Facts: Calories – 215, Total Fat – 13.5g, Saturated Fat – 3.8g, Cholesterol – 27mg, Sodium – 1218mg, Total Carbohydrate – 23.3g, Dietary Fiber – 5.7g, Total Sugars – 11.9g, Protein – 10.9g.

CHAPTER 9: MEAT-BASED - MAIN DISHES

MEATBALLS WITH NOMATO SAUCE

Cook Time: 1 hour

Yield: 12 Meatballs

Ingredients

- 1 lb. of ground beef
- 4 oz. of drained mushrooms
- 1 lb. of ground bison
- Olive oil
- Nomato sauce
- 2 crushed garlic cloves
- ¼ cup of fresh parsley (freshly diced)
- 1 ½ tsp of fine sea salt

Instructions

- Heat your oven to about 350 ºF and set the middle rack in the oven.
- Prepare the baking dish, massage the bottom of the bowl with the olive oil.
- In a large bowl, mix meat, mushrooms, parsley, cloves, and sea salt. It's best to use your hand for proper mixing.
- Scoop out a small portion of the mix (about one-third of a cup) and form it into meatballs.
- Place the meatballs in the prepared baking dish and bake until it is well cooked, and the meat turns brown (usually about 30 – 35 minutes)
- Garnish meatballs with extra parsley and serve with nomato sauce.

Nutrition Facts: Calories – 139, Total Fat – 4.9g, Saturated Fat – 1.5g, Cholesterol – 61mg, Sodium – 401mg, Total Carbohydrate – 0.8g, Dietary Fiber – 0.3g, Total Sugars – 0.1g, Protein – 22g.

SLOW-COOKED DUCK BREAST

Cook Time: 8 hours 10 minutes

Yield: 2 Serves

Ingredients

- 1 lb. of duck breast (diced)
- 2 tsp of cassava flour
- 1 can of coconut milk
- ½ tsp of fine sea salt
- ½ cup of black olives
- ½ tbsp. of oregano
- 1 crushed garlic clove

Instructions

- Prepare a slow cooker and combine all the ingredients in it. Cook for about 8 hours over low heat supply.
- Afterward, remove the meat and olives using a slotted spoon and set aside while kept warm.
- Sprinkle cassava flour over what is left in the slow cooker and mix for 10 – 12 seconds until the sauce

thickens a little. Then, pour the sauce on the meat and serve.

Nutrition Facts: Calories – 1228, Total Fat – 66.6g, Saturated Fat – 28.3g, Cholesterol – 262mg, Sodium – 4426mg, Total Carbohydrate – 31.8g, Dietary Fiber – 2.8g, Total Sugars – 0.3g, Protein – 105.4g.

BALSAMIC-SAUCED CHICKEN LIVERS WITH GRAPES

Cook Time: 32 minutes

Yield: 4 Serves

Ingredients

- 1 pound of chicken livers
- 2 tablespoons of olive oil
- 2 cups of white seedless grapes (halved)
- Fine sea salt to taste
- 2 tablespoons of balsamic vinegar
- ½ cup of pure grape juice
- ½ teaspoon of fine sea salt
- 2 tablespoon of fresh thyme (diced)

The last 4 ingredients are for the sauce

Instructions

- Rinse the chicken livers thoroughly and dry. Remove the white attachments on the livers and cut them into big chunks.

- Place a sizable skillet over medium-high heat. Add the liver chunks and salt to taste. Then cook for about five minutes, flipping the pieces over midways.
- With a spatula, scoop out the meat and set aside.
- Reduce the heat to medium and add the vinegar, grape juice, salt, and thyme. Scrape the bottom of the skillet and mix with the liquid for a minute.
- Then, add the seedless grapes to the skillet, cover-up, and simmer for 7 ½ minutes.
- Remove the heat source, add the livers back to the skillet and mix to be well-coated with the sauce. Then cover and allow to sit for about 5 minutes before serving.

Nutrition Facts: Calories – 423, Total Fat – 14.6g, Saturated Fat – 3.4g, Cholesterol – 638mg, Sodium – 1052mg, Total Carbohydrate – 43g, Dietary Fiber – 0.9g, Total Sugars – 39.6g, Protein – 28.2g.

ELK MEATLOAF WITH APPLE & SAGE

Cook Time: 1 hour 10 minutes

Yield: 1 Serve

Ingredients

- 2 lb. of elk meat
- 1 cup of diced apple
- 2 tbsp. of dried sage
- 1 cup of diced onion
- 4 slices of bacon (diced)
- 2 tsp of fine salt

Instructions

- Heat your oven to about 350 ºF and set the middle rack in the oven. Also, prepare a sizable pan and grease with olive oil.
- Combine all the ingredients in a relatively large bowl and mix well using your hands.
- Evenly press the meat mix into the prepared pan and bake the meatloaf in the preheated oven until meatloaf starts pulling away from the sides of the pan (this usually takes about an hour).

- Serve and enjoy while hot.

Nutrition Facts: Calories – 1600, Total Fat – 55.3g, Saturated Fat – 22.5g, Cholesterol – 767mg, Sodium – 6787mg, Total Carbohydrate – 44.7g, Dietary Fiber – 9.5g, Total Sugars – 28.8g, Protein – 223.4g.

SHALLOTS LAMB ROAST WITH GOLDEN BEETS

Cook Time: 1 hour 35 minutes

Yield: 5 Serves

Ingredients

- 2 pounds leg of lamb (boneless)
- 3 sprigs of fresh rosemary
- 1 tablespoon of olive oil
- 4 garlic cloves
- 4 golden beets (quartered)
- Sea salt to taste
- ¾ lb. of Shallots

Instructions

- Heat the oven to about 350 ºF and set the rack in the middle of the oven.
- Prepare a broiler pan and grease with olive oil.
- Place the lamb (about 2 pounds) at the center of the pan and cut about 12 small unit opening all over the meat.
- Cut the garlic cloves into 3 pieces each (lengthwise) and separate the rosemary leaves from the stem.

- Then, insert one small bunch of rosemary leaves and one piece of garlic into each of the opening made on the meat.

- Nicely arrange the shallots and beets around the meat.

- Add the olive oil, diced rosemary, and salt to taste.

- Roast in the oven for an hour and 15 minutes while occasionally moistening the meat and vegetables. When done, the internal temperature should be about 145 $^{\circ}$F.

- Transfer the lamb roast to a cutting board and allow to cool for 10 minutes before slicing.

Nutrition Facts: Calories – 430, Total Fat – 28.6g, Saturated Fat – 4.1g, Cholesterol – omg, Sodium – 296mg, Total Carbohydrate – 40.4g, Dietary Fiber – 5.8g, Total Sugars – 19.2g, Protein – 7.5g.

CARBONARA SPAGHETTI SQUASH

Cook Time: 1 hour 25 minutes

Yield: 4 Serves

Ingredients

- 1 medium spaghetti squash

- 1 sprig of fresh rosemary

- 1 pound of turkey bacon

- 1 medium onion (yellow)

- 1 cup of black olives (sliced)

- 2 teaspoons of sea salt (divided)

Instructions

- Cut the spaghetti squash in half and remove the seeds. Also, cut the turkey bacon into small pieces and chop the yellow onion.

- Heat up the oven to about 400 °F.

- Add 1 teaspoon of the sea salt to the bottom of the spaghetti squash.

- Combine the turkey bacon, black olive, and onion and divide it into two parts. Fill each part in the center of each halved spaghetti squash and sprinkle the remaining 1 teaspoon of sea salt on it.

- Garnish the squash with pieces of rosemary.

- Get a sizable baking dish and place the two halves of the spaghetti squash on the dish.

- Put on the middle rack in the oven and allow to bake for an hour. Serve hot.

Nutrition Facts: Calories – 672, Total Fat – 51.2g, Saturated Fat – 16.1g, Cholesterol – 125mg, Sodium – 3854mg, Total Carbohydrate – 8.1g, Dietary Fiber – 1.7g, Total Sugars – 1.2g, Protein – 42.8g.

ROSEMARY AND PEARS ROASTED CHICKEN

Cook Time: 1 hour 15 minutes

Yield: Varies

Ingredients

- 1 whole chicken

- 1 tablespoon of olive oil

- Extra olive oil for the dish

- 3 sprigs of fresh rosemary

- 3 Bartlett pears

- 1 teaspoon of salt

Instructions

- Cut chicken in pieces and grease the cooking dish with the extra olive oil.

- Heat up the oven to about 350 ºF.

- Place the chicken pieces in the cooking dish (avoid overlapping) and sprinkle with salt.

- Also, cut the pears in 4 pieces and remove the seeds. Place the pieces around the meat in the dish and add a little fresh rosemary over the meat.

- Drizzle olive oil on the chicken and cook in the preheated oven for about an hour.

- For better results, baste the chicken with cooking juices at two different intervals.

Nutrition Facts: Calories – 162, Total Fat – 5g, Saturated Fat – 0.7g, Cholesterol – 0mg, Sodium – 778mg, Total Carbohydrate – 32g, Dietary Fiber – 6.6g, Total Sugars – 20.4g, Protein – 0.8g.

CROCKPOT CHICKEN WITH CARROTS & APPLES

Cook Time: 8 hours 10 minutes

Yield: 6 Serves

Ingredients

- 2 pounds of chicken breasts

- 2 ½ apples (roughly diced)

- 5 big carrots

- 1 can of coconut milk

- 1 ½ onion (roughly diced)

- 10 pitted plums

- 2 teaspoons of salt

- Fresh Sage (diced)

Instructions

- Prepare a slow cooker. Cut the chicken breasts into big chunks and arrange at the bottom of the slow cooker

- Add carrots, onions, and apples with the apples being on top. Add the ten plums and pour the coconut milk all over the ingredients.

- Then, cook the mix for about 8 hours inside the slow cooker on low heat.

- When the contents of the crockpot are about to be done, add salt to taste and toss all the ingredients together to be well mixed.

- When done, serve with a sprinkle of fresh sage.

Nutrition Facts: Calories – 514, Total Fat – 21.3g, Saturated Fat – 11.6g, Cholesterol – 135mg, Sodium – 954mg, Total Carbohydrate – 37.1g, Dietary Fiber – 6.8g, Total Sugars – 26.8g, Protein – 46.6g.

DAIRY-FREE ALFREDO CHICKEN

Cook Time:

Yield: 2 Serves

Ingredients

- ¾ lb. of chicken breasts (boneless and skinless)

- 1 zucchini

- Sea Salt to taste

- Crushed fresh parsley

- 1 cup of chicken broth

- 2 tsp of nutritional yeast

- 1 ½ tbsp. of arrowroot flour

- 1 cup of coconut milk

- 1 tsp of dried basil

- 1 tsp of garlic powder

- ½ tsp of fine sea salt

Instructions

- Cut both ends of zucchini and then cut in half.

- Make the zucchini into noodles using a spiralizer and keep aside.

- Using a paper towel, dry the chicken breasts, and sprinkle salt on both sides.

- Prepare a skillet and heat the coconut oil in it over medium heat.

- Add chicken to the oil and cook for about 8 minutes or until it's no longer pink inside (internal temperature should be 165 °F).

- Place the chicken on a cutting board. Allow to cool for two – three minutes before cutting into strips (about ½ inch in thickness).

- Whisk together the broth and arrowroot flour in a bowl, ensuring there are no flour lumps.

- In the same skillet, combine coconut milk, yeast, basil, garlic, and salt. Bring the mix to a boil with medium heat.

- Add the broth mixture into the skillet and adjust the heat to medium-low. Stir consistently for about 2 minutes till the sauce thickens a little. Check if more seasoning is needed and adjust if necessary. Then, add the zucchini noodles to the skillet and toss around to coat the noodles with the sauce.

- Serve noodles with sliced chicken on top and garnish with crushed parsley. Enjoy.

Nutrition Facts: Calories – 656, Total Fat – 42.3g, Saturated Fat – 29.1g, Cholesterol – 151mg, Sodium – 679mg, Total Carbohydrate – 14g, Dietary Fiber – 5g, Total Sugars – 6.4g, Protein – 57.7g.

CHAPTER 10: SEAFOOD RECIPES

OYSTER SAUERKRAUT SOUP

Cook Time: 20 minutes

Yield: 4 Serves

Ingredients

- 24 oz. of sauerkraut

- 16 oysters (out of shell)

- Sea salt to taste

- 4 cups of bone broth or water

- 1 tbsp. of green onion (diced)

Instructions

- Thoroughly rinse the sauerkraut with cold water to reduce the sourness.

- Prepare a large pot, add bone broth (or water) to it and bring to a boil.

- Add oysters to the pot and bring to a boil again. Keep boiling the mix for about 5 minutes

- Add salt to taste

- Garnish with the diced green onions when serving.

Nutrition Facts: Calories – 204, Protein – 20g, Fat – 6g, Carbohydrates – 15g, Fiber – 3g, Sugar – 2g.

SHRIMP FRIED CAULIFLOWER RICE

Cook Time: 25 minutes

Yield: 2 Serves

Ingredients

- ½ pound of shrimp (peeled)

- 2 garlic cloves (diced)

- 1 head of cauliflower

- 2 carrots (diced)

- 1 medium onion (diced)

- 2 green onions (diced)

- 4 tbsp. of avocado oil

- 2 tbsp. of coconut aminos

- Salt to taste

Instructions

- Peel the shrimp and break the cauliflower into florets. Dry cauliflower and squeeze out excess water.

- Prepare a saucepan, put avocado oil in the pan and cook the peeled shrimp, garlic cloves and diced onion in it until onions turn brown and shrimp is cooked.

- Remove from the saucepan and set aside.

- Process the florets in a food processor until the consistency of small rice-looking pieces.

- Add the cauliflower rice and carrots to the saucepan and cook until they are softened.

- Put the shrimp, garlic, and onions back in the saucepan, top with the green onions and season with salt to taste and coconut aminos. Serve.

Nutrition Facts: Calories – 482, Protein – 29g, Fat – 31g, Carbohydrates – 27g, Sugar – 12g, Fiber – 9g.

COCONUT SHRIMP AND GRITS

Cook Time: 25 minutes

Yield: 4 Serves

Ingredients

- 9 ounces of uncooked shrimp (peeled)

- 2 tbsp. of olive oil

- 15 button mushrooms (chopped)

- 2 garlic cloves (crushed)

- 1 cup of coconut cream

- Salt to taste

- $2/3$ cup of desiccated coconut (unsweetened)

- Lemon juice

- 2 tbsp. of diced flat-leaf parsley (if desired)

Instructions

- Prepare a frying pan, add olive oil, and sauté the mushrooms for about 5 minutes.

- Add the shrimp and cook until pink. Add the squeezed lemon juice and salt to taste, then set aside.

- Heat the unsweetened coconut inside the coconut cream to make the grits.

- Serve the shrimp mix on the grits and garnish with parsley if desired.

Nutrition Facts: Calories – 328, Sugar – 3g, Protein – 13g, Fat – 28g, Carbohydrates – 7g, Fiber – 3g.

COCONUT SHRIMP LIME

Cook Time: 10 minutes

Yield: 2 Serves

Ingredients

- 7 ounces of shrimp

- 2 tbsp. of coconut flour

- Coconut oil

- ½ cup of coconut flakes

- Salt

- Lime wedges

Instructions

- Prepare a bowl, combine the coconut flour and coconut flakes in the bowl.

- Add the shrimp and press the coconut into the shrimp nicely.

- Deep-fry the shrimp in coconut oil for a couple of minutes (using a slotted spoon to put the shrimps in the oil).

- Remove the shrimps with the slotted spoon and transfer to a tray lined with a paper towel.

- Season with salt and lime. Serve and enjoy while warm.

Nutrition Facts: Calories – 223, Protein – 22g, Fat – 13g, Sugar – 2g, Carbohydrates – 7g, Fiber – 4g.

SALMON NORI WRAP

Cook Time: 10 minutes

Yield: 2 wraps

Ingredients

- 1 large avocado (sliced)

- 2 Nori sheets

- 5 $\frac{1}{3}$ ounces of smoked salmon

- Cilantro

- ¼ carrot (peeled and sliced)

- 1 green onion (sliced)

Instructions

- Peel the carrot and slice thinly. Also, slice the avocado thinly.

- Run your finger under water and gently wipe the nori sheets all over with your damp finger - to dampen the nori wraps.

- Then, lay the avocado, carrots, smoked salmon, and green onion on the nori. Sprinkle cilantro on the nori to garnish (this is optional).

- Roll up the nori wrap and relish.

Nutrition Facts: Calories per wrap – 261, Protein – 16g, Fat – 17g, Fiber – 8g, Sugar – 1g, Carbohydrates – 10g.

AIP-FRIENDLY CEVICHE

Cook Time: 40 minutes

Yield: 2 Serves

Ingredients

- 1½ fillets of fresh white fish

- 1½ Limes (juiced)

- ½ avocado (peeled and diced)

- ¼ red onion (finely diced)

- 2 tbsp. of cilantro (finely diced)

- Salt to taste

Instructions

- Ensure the white fish is skinless and deboned. Cut the fish into half-inch pieces.

- In a bowl, mix up the fish, red onion, and juice from the limes.

- After mixing well, cover-up, and refrigerate for 30 minutes - do not refrigerate for more than 30 minutes.

- Stir in the avocado and cilantro (parsley can be used as an alternative) and season with salt before serving.

Nutrition Facts: Calories – 195, protein – 23g, Fat – 9g, Sugar – 2g, Carbohydrates – 7g, Fiber – 4g.

SMOKED SALMON CEVICHE

Cook Time: 10 minutes

Yield: 1 Serve

Ingredients

- 78g of smoked salmon (roughly diced)

- ½ lime

- ½ large avocado (peeled and diced)

- Cilantro (finely diced)

Instructions

- Toss the smoked salmon together with the diced avocado in a dish.

- Squeeze the lime over the dish and sprinkle the finely diced cilantro to garnish.

- Serve and enjoy.

Nutrition Facts: Calories – 256, Protein – 16g, Fat – 17g, Carbohydrates – 10g, Fiber – 7g, Sugar – 2g.

FISH BONE BROTH

Cook Time: 4 hours 5 minutes

Yield: 6 – 8 Serves

Ingredients

- Fish head

- 4 slices of ginger

- Water

- 1 tbsp. of lemon juice

- Salt to taste

- ½ leek (sliced)

Instructions

- Pour cold water in a large pot and put the fish head in the pot. Bring to a boil and drain the water away.

- Fill the pot with fresh water and add the lemon juice, leek, ginger, and sea salt to taste.

- Then simmer for about 4 hours with the lid.

Nutrition Facts: Calories – 40, Protein – 5g, Carbohydrate – 0g, Sugar – 0g, Fat – 2g, Fiber – 0g.

NOMATO-SAUCED SHRIMP

Cook Time: 10 minutes

Yield: 2 Serves

Ingredients

- 7 ounces of Shrimp (peeled and cooked)

- 2 tbsp. of Nomato Ketchup

- Salt

- 1 cup of shredded iceberg lettuce

- 2 tbsp. of coconut cream

- Lemon wedges

- Avocado slices and Parsley to garnish

Instructions

- Mix the Nomato ketchup with the coconut cream and add salt to taste.

- Add the Shrimp to the mix and toss together to ensure shrimp is well coated.

- Put the shredded lettuce in a bowl and place the shrimp on it. Squeeze the lemon over the shrimp and garnish with avocado and parsley.

- Serve immediately.

Nutrition Facts: Calories – 132, Fat – 5g, Protein – 20g, Carbohydrate – 1g, Fiber – 1g, Sugar – 0g. (Ketchup excluded from nutritional facts).

STUFFED SALMON WITH CRAB

Cook Time: 30 minutes

Yield: 1 – 2 Serves

Ingredients

- ½ pound of Salmon fillet

- 1 piece of turkey bacon

- Olive oil

- 2 ounces of cooked crab meat (canned)

- 2 tablespoons of parsley (diced)

- 1 lime (juiced)

Instructions

- Heat your oven to about 200 °C.

- Prepare a baking dish and line with parchment paper.

- Cook the turkey bacon and set aside.

- For the stuffing, mix crab with parsley, turkey bacon, lime juice, and olive oil.

- Carefully slice the salmon down the middle, not getting deep through the skin.

- Fill the slit with the prepared stuffing and place it in a baking pan.

- Bake for 20 minutes or until salmon is well cooked.

- Then broil for about 5 minutes or until the salmon's top is brown.

Nutrition Facts: Calories – 365, Total Fat – 25.6g, Saturated Fat – 7.8g, Cholesterol – 89mg, Sodium – 471mg, Total Carbohydrate – 4.4g, Dietary Fiber – 1.1g, Total Sugars – 0.6g, Protein – 29.4g.

CHAPTER 11: DESSERT RECIPES

AMBROSIA SALAD

Cook Time: 5 minutes

Yield: 4 Serves

Ingredients

- 1 cup of coconut cream

- 3 ½ ounces of fresh raspberries

- 3 ½ ounces of fresh blackberries

- 3 ½ ounces of fresh pineapple, diced

- 3 ½ ounces of fresh blueberries

- 2 tbsp. of shredded coconut

Instructions

- Using a mixer or a whisk, whip the coconut cream until it is slightly thick.

- In a bowl, add all the fresh berries and the pineapple together and stir gently.

- Serve in 4 dish bowls and garnish with the shredded coconut (optional).

Nutrition Facts: Calories – 187, Sugar – 10g, Protein – 0g, Fat – 14g, Carbohydrate – 16g, Fiber – 5g.

CHOCOLATE-LIKE COOKIES

Cook Time: 25 minutes

Yield: 8 Serves

Ingredients

- ¾ cup of Carob Powder

- 10 tbsp. of coconut flour

- ¼ cup of cassava flour

- 3 tbsp. of coconut oil

- 2 tbsp. of water

- 5 tbsp. of honey

- Extra hot water

- 1 tbsp. of agar agar powder

Instructions

- Heat your oven to about 180 °C.

- Mix agar agar powder with water in a sizable bowl. Bring the mixture to a boil and allow to simmer for a few minutes, stirring until dissolved.

- In a separate bowl, mix the coconut flour, carob powder, and cassava flour in it.

- In another bowl, whisk the prepared agar agar together with the honey.

- Then, add the wet mix to the dry mix and add the extra hot water. Combine well using a spoon.

- Form small sized balls (about an ounce) from the dough mix and place each ball on a baking dish or a tray lined with parchment paper.

- Gently press down on the balls to form the shape of a cookie and put the dish or tray into the preheated oven for 15 minutes.

- Remove cookies and allow to cool for 15 minutes before serving.

Nutrition Facts: Calories – 123, Protein – 2g, Sugar – 8g, Fat – 6g, Carbohydrate – 15g, Fiber – 3g.

MARSHMALLOWS

Cook Time: 30 minutes

Yield: 10 Serves

Ingredients

- 3 tbsp. of agar agar powder

- Avocado oil

- ½ cup of cold water

- 1/3 cup of honey

- ½ cup of warm water

- Carob powder (if desired, for dusting)

Instructions

- Prepare a sizable pan and line with parchment paper. Apply avocado oil on the parchment paper.

- Mix agar agar powder with cold water in a sizable bowl. Bring the mixture to a boil and allow to simmer for a few minutes, stirring until dissolved.

- In a pot, pour water and honey into it. Heat until well mixed (avoid boiling for a long time).

- Using an electric whisk or a stand mixer, whisk the agar agar mix slowly at first then increase the whisking speed. Gently add the hot honey mix to the mixing bowl and keep whisking for about 10 minutes (mixture should be creamy and white).

- Thicken the mixture by whisking for an additional 10 minutes until the mixture doubles and looks like marshmallow fluff.

- Then, pour the mixture into the prepared pan already lined with greased parchment paper. Then put in the fridge for 5 – 6 hours.

- If desired, dust with carob powder or arrowroot powder. Cut and serve.

Nutrition Facts: Calories – 23, Protein – 2g, Fat – 0g, Sugar – 4g, Fiber – 0g, Carbohydrates – 5g.

MILK POPSICLES

Cook Time: 5 minutes

Yield: 4 Serves

Ingredients

- 1 cup of coconut milk

- 2 tbsp. of raw honey

- 1 tsp of ground ginger

- ½ tbsp. of turmeric powder

- Cinnamon

Instructions

- Prepare a saucepan and add in coconut milk and honey. Heat slightly. Spice it up by adding the spices and, if desired, add more honey to the mix.

- Then, divide the mix into popsicle molds and refrigerate for about 4 hours.

- Serve

Nutrition Facts: Calories – 131, Protein – 1g, Fat – 11g, Fiber – 0g, Sugar – 6g, Carbohydrates – 8g.

WAFFLES WITH PUMPKIN SPICE

Cook Time: 15 minutes

Yield: 2 Serves

Ingredients

- 2 tsp of beef gelatin

- 1 cup of cassava flour

- 2 tbsp. of hot water

- ½ tsp of baking soda

- ½ tsp of cream of tartar

- Salt

- 2 tbsp. of pumpkin puree

- 1½ tsp of reserved pumpkin spice

- 1½ tbsp. of coconut oil (melted)

- 2 tbsp. of honey

- ½ cup of boiling water

- ½ tsp of ground cinnamon

- ½ tbsp. of ground ginger

- Ground mace

The last 3 ingredients are for the pumpkin spice

Instructions

- Combine all the ingredients for the pumpkin spice together in a container and place it aside.

- Add the gelatin powder to 2 tbsp. of hot water in another container and place it aside as well.

- Combine cassava flour, baking soda, salt, the cream of tartar, and pumpkin spice in a mixing bowl.

- Get a separate bowl and whisk together the pumpkin puree, honey, and melted oil. Stir in the gelatin mixture and the boiling water.

- Mix to combine; then, add the dry mixture. Continue to stir until the desired thick slurry consistency is achieved (add more boiling water if required).

- Grease a waffle maker and heat up. Add the flour mix and cook waffles until crispy.

- When done, remove gently, drizzle with honey, and serve hot.

Nutrition Facts: Calories – 367, Sugar – 12g, Protein – 3g, Fiber – 5g, Fat – 9g, Carbohydrates – 70g.

CREAM COCONUT PIE

Cook Time: 30 minutes

Yield: 8 Serves

Ingredients

- 2 tsp of beef gelatin

- 1½ cups of coconut flour

- 2½ tbsp. of honey

- 2 tbsp. of hot water for the filling

- 2½ tbsp. of coconut oil (melted)

- 1 cup of coconut cream

- 6 tbsp. of hot water for the base

- ¼ cup of honey

- ¼ cup of coconut milk (full fat)

Instructions

- Heat your oven to about 180 ºC.

- Whisk together the coconut oil, honey, and hot water in a bowl and put the coconut flour in a separate bowl.

- Add the wet mix to the bowl containing the flour and work the mixture until it looks like breadcrumbs.

- Prepare a pie dish, pour the mixture into the dish and press down into an even compact layer.

- Bake the mix in the preheated oven for 8 minutes. Turn off the oven and leave in the oven for another 10 minutes, then remove and allow to cool.

- Dissolve the gelatin powder into the hot water and set aside.

- Whisk together the coconut milk and the coconut cream until the mix is free of lumps. Add honey to the mix and the gelatin mixture, then stir well to combine.

- Pour the filling on the crust and refrigerate for 4 hours before serving.

Nutrition Facts: Calories – 210, Protein – 4g, Sugar – 11g, Fat -13g, Fiber – 6g, Carbohydrates – 18g.

BERRY MIX CRUMBLE

Cook Time: 35 minutes

Yield: 6 Serves

Ingredients

- 40 oz. of mixed berries

- 1 tbsp. of lemon juice

- 6 tbsp. of cassava flour

- 3 tbsp. of coconut oil

- 6½ tbsp.. of coconut flour

- ¾ cup of shredded coconut

Instructions

- Heat your oven to about 180 °C.

- Put all the berries in a mixing bowl, add lemon juice and gently squish the berries. Stir well and divide the berries between 6 fireproof ramekins placed on a tray and placed in the preheated oven to bake for about 20 minutes.

- While baking, cut the coconut oil into small pieces and combine with cassava flour and coconut flour in a bowl.

- Work the mixture until it looks like coarse breadcrumbs. Add the shredded coconut into the mix and stir well.

- After baking the berries mix, remove the tray from the oven and evenly spread the crumb-like mixture over the six fireproof ramekins, then put the tray back into the oven and allow it to cook for another 8 minutes.

- When it is done, the top will be golden and crispy

- Serve or garnish with extra coconut before serving (if desired).

Nutrition Facts: Calories – 436, Protein – 2g, Fat – 14g, Fiber – 32g, Sugar – 32g, Carbohydrates – 76g.

COCONUT CASSAVA PANCAKES

Cook Time: 35 minutes

Yield: 3 Serves

Ingredients

- 1½ tbsp. of beef gelatin

- ¾ cup of coconut flour

- 3 tbsp. of hot water

- Cinnamon

- ½ cup of cassava flour

- ½ cup of coconut milk (warm)

- 2 tbsp. of coconut oil

- 4 tbsp. of honey

- Berries

Instructions

- To prepare gelatin, sprinkle the powder over a small bowl containing the hot water and allow to dissolve and mix well, then set it aside.

- In a bowl, combine the cassava flour, coconut flour, and a dash of cinnamon together.

- Add the gelatin mixture, the warm coconut milk, and honey to the bowl and whisk together, ensuring there is no lump in the mix.

- Get a relatively larger bowl and pour hot water in it, put the bowl containing the mixture in hot water to keep the mix warm.

- Over medium heat, add small coconut oil to a pan. Scoop out about ¼ of a cup of the batter from the mixture and spread it out by turning the pan around.

- Then, allow the pancake to cook for about 4 minutes, flip over the pancake gently using a large spatula. Cook on the underside for about 3 more minutes.

- Next, transfer onto a prepared plate lined with kitchen paper (this will absorb excess coconut oil). Drizzle with honey.

- Repeat the process for the remaining coconut oil and batter.

- Serve pancakes warm with berries.

Nutrition Facts: Calories – 349, Protein – 8g, Fat – 14g, Fiber – 11g, Sugar – 17g, Carbohydrates – 46g.

BROWNIE BITES (RAW)

Cook Time: 10 minutes

Yield: 1 Serve

Ingredients:

- ¼ cup of shredded coconut (unsweetened)

- 14 ounces of soft dates

- 3 tbsp. of melted coconut oil

- 3 tbsp. of carob powder

Instructions

- Prepare a mini food processor, place the melted coconut oil, soft dates, and carob powder in it and run until the mixture is well combined.

- Prepare a tray lined with parchment paper and scrape out the mass on the tray.

- Flatten the mixture into a fairly sizeable compact square using the back of a metal spoon.

- Spread the shredded coconut all over the mixture and press it into the surface gently.

- Place the tray into the fridge and refrigerate for 20 minutes.

- Remove from the fridge and slice the mixture into small 1-inch squares.

- Serve immediately or put back in the fridge to eat later.

Nutrition Facts: Calories – 70, Protein – 0g, Sugar – 12g, Fat – 2g, Fiber – 2g, Carbohydrates – 14g.

COCONUT POPSICLES

Cook Time: 10 minutes

Yield: 2 Serves

Ingredients

- ¼ cup of coconut milk

- 1 tsp of raw honey

- ½ cup of blueberries

- 1 tbsp. of lemon juice

- Salt

Instructions

- Using a blender, blend all the ingredients.

- Transfer the mixture into ice pop molds, ensuring that there is room for expansion when popsicle freezes.

- Then, freeze for several hours (about 4 – 5 hours)

- Before serving, place ice pop mold under hot water for a couple of minutes to ease up the ice pops and make it easier to pull.

Nutrition Facts: Calories – 102, Protein – 1g, Sugar – 7g, Fat – 7g, Sodium – 11mg, Carbohydrates – 10g.

CONCLUSION

The Autoimmune protocol is all about controlling your diet to achieve better health. While being diagnosed with an autoimmune disease can be a lot, a significant way of restoring your health is the Autoimmune Protocol Diet. It is impressive how the diet-based approach works in the restoration and balancing of the body systems. AIP is designed to be a short-term healing approach. Although, many people may choose to continue with this diet after the symptoms of the autoimmune disorders had gone. The AIP diet allows the use of vegetables (except nightshades), fruits, proteins, and healthy fats. It hammers on staying away from gluten, grains, dairy products, soy, legumes, nightshades, eggs, food additives, nuts, and seeds. This is because gluten is inflammatory to the gut. At the same time, grains and legumes produce anti-nutrients like inflammatory lectins and phytic acid, artificial sugar and alcohol are also highly inflammatory, and they interfere with the healing process, nightshade vegetables are known to be inflammatory. They lead to gut discomfort; food additives have no known health benefits but are known to be pro-inflammatory and allergenic. It is essential to avoid all these and follow the strict eating plan of the AIP diet to achieve the desired result within the short time frame.

After following the AIP diet for the recommended period, reintroducing foods can be a little tricky, and it is crucial to be guided during this period. The idea is to avoid reintroducing many foods at a time; it is recommended to start with one new food per time and study how your body reacts for about 2 – 3 days. It is advisable to keep a journal for this purpose and then identify foods that work and the ones that do not work while repeating the process of one meal at a time.

How to know if healing has taken place and the AIP diet has finally worked is quite different between individuals; however, the pointers would be a noticeable reduction in the initial symptoms and a change in blood work. As stated earlier in this guide, to achieve a better result with the AIP diet, it is essential to support this diet with a healthy lifestyle practice. This involves getting enough sleep, reducing stress, working with your health coach to keep track of your journey, and also staying active. Although the AIP diet is a significant part of the healing process, complete healing usually takes more than just following the diet alone. It is vital to embrace a healthy lifestyle practice to compliment the AIP diet.

Listed below are some terms used in the recipes provided in this guide to aid a better understanding. Keep in mind that all Nutrition Facts contained in this guide are estimated values and are based on the amount per serve.

1. **Parchment Paper:** This is an already coated cellulose-based paper used in baking. The coating makes it non-sticky.

2. **Food Processor:** This is an appliance, similar to a blender, which is used to dice, chop, blend, and slice food to aid faster meal preparation.

3. **Crispy:** This is a condition of being tender and brittle.

4. **Broil:** To broil means to cook by direct exposure to heat (an oven or a part of the stove is usually used for broiling).

5. **Simmer:** This means to boil slowly at low temperature.

6. **Slow cooker:** Slow cooker or a crock-pot is used to simmer at low temperature

7. **Headspace:** This is the distance between the surface of the food in the jar and the underside of the jar lid.

8. **Sauté:** This means to fry quickly in a little fat or to fry briefly over high heat supply.

In conclusion, it should be noted that the autoimmune protocol is not exactly a cure for autoimmune diseases, but it works impressively in reversing the symptoms caused by these diseases. Staying on the AIP diet for the recommended period, optimizing your nutrient intake, taking a careful systematic approach when reintroducing foods into your diet, and embracing a healthy lifestyle practice are ways of getting the best out of the autoimmune protocol.

OTHER BOOKS BY HOLLY KRISTIN

Ayurveda Cookbook

https://mybook.to/HollyKristinAyurveda

Baked Donut Cookbook

http://mybook.to/hollykristinbakeddonut

Pressure Canning Cookbook

https://mybook.to/HollyKristinCanning

Mediterranean Diet Cookbook

https://mybook.to/HollyKristinMedDiet

Rheumatoid Arthritis Cookbook

http://getbook.at/hollykristinrheumatoid

Canning & Preserving for Beginners

https://mybook.to/HollyKristinPreserving

The Essential Wood Pellet Smoker and Grill Cookbook

https://getbook.at/woodpelletcookbook

Made in the USA
Las Vegas, NV
04 January 2024

83916527R00125